60 HIKES WITHIN 60 MILES

NASHVILLE

INCLUDING **Clarksville, Gallatin, Murfreesboro,** and the BEST of **Middle Tennessee**

FOURTH EDITION

D0107536

Johnny Molloy

MENASHA RIDGE PRESS
Birmingham, Alabama

60 Hikes Within 60 Miles: Nashville

Copyright © 2016 by Johnny Molloy
All rights reserved
Printed in the United States of America
Published by Menasha Ridge Press
Distributed by Publishers Group West
Fourth edition, first printing

Library of Congress Cataloging-in-Publication Data

Names: Molloy, Johnny, 1961-
Title: 60 hikes within 60 miles, Nashville : including Clarksville, Columbia,
    Gallatin, and Murfreesboro / Johnny Molloy.
Description: Fourth edition. | Birmingham : Menasha Ridge Press, [2016] |
    "Distributed by Publishers Group West"—T.p. verso. | Includes index.
Identifiers: LCCN 2015045306| ISBN 9781634040624 | ISBN 9781634040631 (eBook)
Subjects: LCSH: Hiking—Tennessee—Nashville Region—Guidebooks. |
    Trails—Tennessee—Nashville Region—Guidebooks. | Nashville Region
    (Tenn.) —Guidebooks.
Classification: LCC GV199.42.T22 N376 2016 | DDC 796.5109768/55—dc23
LC record available at http://lccn.loc.gov/2015045306

Cover design: Scott McGrew
Text design: Annie Long
Maps: Scott McGrew and Johnny Molloy
Cover photo © Dennis Hardley/Alamy Stock Photo
Cover and interior photos by Johnny Molloy unless otherwise noted

MENASHA RIDGE PRESS
An imprint of AdventureKEEN
2204 First Ave. S, Ste. 102
Birmingham, AL 35233

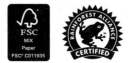

Visit **menasharidge.com** for a complete listing of our books and for ordering information. Contact us at our website, at **facebook.com/menasharidge**, at **twitter.com/menasharidge**, or at **blog.menasharidge.com** with questions or comments.

DISCLAIMER

This book is meant only as a guide to select trails in the Nashville area and does not guarantee hiker safety in any way—you hike at your own risk. Neither Menasha Ridge Press nor Johnny Molloy is liable for property loss or damage, personal injury, or death that result in any way from accessing or hiking the trails described in the following pages. Please be aware that hikers have been injured in the Nashville area. Be especially cautious when walking on or near boulders, steep inclines, and drop-offs, and do not attempt to explore terrain that may be beyond your abilities. To help ensure an uneventful hike, please read carefully the introduction to this book, and perhaps get further safety information and guidance from other sources. Familiarize yourself thoroughly with the areas you intend to visit before venturing out. Ask questions, and prepare for the unforeseen. Familiarize yourself with current weather reports, maps of the area you intend to visit, and any relevant park regulations.

THIS BOOK IS DEDICATED TO THE PEOPLE OF NASHVILLE AND MIDDLE TENNESSEE, WHETHER THEY ARE NATIVES, TRANSPLANTS, OR JUST HERE TO PLAY MUSIC.

Overview Map Key

Other cities in the 60 Hikes Within 60 Miles series:

Albuquerque

Atlanta

Baltimore

Boston

Chicago

Cincinnati

Cleveland

Dallas and Fort Worth

Denver and Boulder

Harrisburg

Houston

Los Angeles

Madison

Minneapolis and St. Paul

New York City

Philadelphia

Phoenix

Pittsburgh

Portland

Richmond

Sacramento

Salt Lake City

San Antonio and Austin

San Diego

San Francisco

Seattle

St. Louis

Washington, D.C.

Table of Contents

Acknowledgments

I WOULD LIKE TO THANK many people for helping me with this project: Keri Anne Molloy, Kelly Stewart and the Nashville Hiking Meetup Group, Carl Nelson and Michael Nelson, Pam Morgan, Dave Gilfillan, Lisa Daniel, Bud Zehmer (for coming up with the idea for the book), and Matt and Bailey Fields. I'd also like to thank Russell Helms, the rangers of Tennessee State Parks (including but not limited to John Froeschauer, Ben Myers, Tim Burris, Shane Petty, Amy Atkins, and Connie of Lebanon), the personnel at the Army Corps of Engineers lakes of Middle Tennessee, and the folks at the Natchez Trace Parkway. And thanks to Diane Manas of the Tennessee Trails Association and everyone I met on the trail.

—*Johnny Molloy*

Foreword

WELCOME TO MENASHA RIDGE PRESS'S 60 Hikes Within 60 Miles, a series designed to provide hikers with the information they need to find and hike the very best trails surrounding metropolitan areas typically underserved by outdoor guidebooks.

Our strategy was simple: First, find a hiker who knows the area and loves to hike. Second, ask that person to spend a year researching the most popular and very best trails around. And third, have that person describe each trail in terms of difficulty, scenery, condition, and all other categories of information that are important to hikers. "Pretend you've just completed a hike and met up with other hikers at the trailhead," we told each author. "Imagine their questions; be clear in your answers."

An experienced hiker and writer, author Johnny Molloy has selected 60 of the best hikes in and around the Nashville metropolitan area. From the rail trails and urban hikes that make use of parklands and streets, to flora- and fauna-rich treks along the numerous area lakes and hills in the hinterlands, to aerobic outings in the mountains, Molloy provides both hikers and walkers with a great variety of hikes—all within roughly 60 miles of Nashville.

You'll get more out of this book if you take a moment to read the Introduction explaining how to read the trail listings. The "Maps" section will help you understand how useful topos will be on a hike and will tell you where to get them. And though this is a where-to, not a how-to, guide, experienced hikers and novices alike will find the Introduction of particular value.

As much for the opportunity to free the spirit as to free the body, let Johnny Molloy's hikes elevate you above the urban hurry.

All the best,
The Editors at Menasha Ridge Press

Preface

WELCOME TO THE FOURTH EDITION OF *60 Hikes Within 60 Miles: Nashville.* The state of hiking in metro Music City continues to improve. New trails—included in this book— have been constructed and greenways expanded. Beyond hiking, Nashville is best known as the capital of country music and of Tennessee. Situated in the Cumberland River Valley and surrounded by hills of the Highland Rim, Nashville and its environs are nothing if not historic. In fact, most of the trails included in this guidebook have a historic bent, allowing visitors to walk both in nature and back in time.

Nashville's first citizens floated to the location on flatboats from East Tennessee. They headed down the Tennessee River, then up the Ohio and Cumberland Rivers to reach the area that would become the city, which is located near a large riverside flat where American Indians had been living for years. Simultaneously, long hunters (early pioneers who went on extended hikes) penetrated the basin from the east to find plentiful game attracted by the area's natural salt licks.

Early in its history, Nashville became the northern terminus of the Natchez Trace, a historic American Indian trace, or trail, between the city and Natchez, Mississippi. In the early 1800s, boatmen walked north from Natchez after floating their crops and goods downriver from the Cumberland River Valley, the Ohio River Valley, and points north. Later, simple farmers settled in the Nashville Basin, opening what was then the west by clearing fields and building walls of stone that are now a Middle Tennessee hallmark.

Modern Middle Tennessee history begins in the Nashville settlement. Old Stone Fort State Park, near Manchester, houses a paleo-Indian site where the ancients built a wall. The reason it was built remains a mystery to this day. You can visit the wall for yourself and try to come up with a theory. And near Hohenwald, you can walk to the very spot where heralded American explorer Meriwether Lewis spent his last night on Earth at Grinder's Stand. There's evidence of the establishment of early Tennessee industry at Montgomery Bell's iron-forge site in Dickson County. And Johnsonville State Historic Park, to the west in Humphreys County, is the location of Nathan Bedford Forrest's unprecedented defeat of a naval force by a cavalry during the Civil War.

Dunbar Cave, up Clarksville way, held old-time hoedowns led by none other than country music icon Roy Acuff. And other trails in Maury County preserve remnants of the original Natchez Trace built 200 years ago. You can walk these trails today and follow the footsteps of untold thousands who tramped by foot and horseback along Middle Tennessee's first "interstate," which is now preserved as a recreational hiking trail.

Some area parks have been created to memorialize both history and nature. The establishment of the Warner Parks and Radnor Lake State Park, for instance, recall stories of early citizen action aimed at preserving our natural heritage decades ago. Bowie Nature Park, near Fairview, tells the tale of three sisters who turned a worn-out family farm into a restored nature habitat.

Middle Tennessee is also laced with man-made lakes. Mostly built in the last half century, these impoundments were established for flood control and commerce on the Cumberland and Tennessee river systems. These lakes have created recreational opportunities, such as boating, swimming, and fishing. With the establishment of Tennessee state parks and Army Corps of Engineers recreation areas on their shorelines, they have also become hiking destinations. Long Hunter State Park, on Percy Priest Lake, has many trails traversing the lakeshore and passing through interesting habitats, including rock gardens and cedar woods. Other areas, such as Newsome's Mill, were once settled and now preserve the relics of a former community.

The fast-growing Old Hickory Lake area has trails, too, such as the loop hike at Bledsoe Creek State Park that offers new residents nature getaways as Nashville expands ever outward. There are remote places, such as the Wilderness Trail, that cover some of the roughest terrain in Middle Tennessee, along the steep shoreline of Cordell Hull Lake in Jackson County. And Fort Donelson National Battlefield stands tall on the shoreline of Lake Barkley, offering insights into Civil War battle strategies.

You can't forget the rivers. Tennessee's waterways have always been travel corridors, and now they're also hiking corridors. The Eagle Trail rises above the Caney Fork River. The Old Mill Trail bordering the Duck River explores a historic river ford used by Andrew Jackson and is the site of a corn-grinding station once run by a Tennessee governor. And the Narrows of Harpeth Trail climbs to a vista overlooking the lower Harpeth River. Smaller streams—such as Spring Creek at Sellars Farm State Archaeological Area and Vaughn's Creek on the Harpeth Woods Trail—are also worth exploring. And many other unnamed creeks can be seen and crossed on other hikes.

Of course, some areas have been established and preserved purely for their overall scenic or natural beauty. Short Springs State Natural Area is set aside primarily for its waterfalls and wildflowers. Flat Rock Cedar Glades and Barrens harbors rare plants unique to Middle Tennessee. Beaman Park preserves the oak ridges and steep-sided, wildflower-carpeted valleys of the Highland Rim. And Devil's Backbone State Natural Area harbors an intact hickory–oak upland forest with little intrusion from nonnative plants and animals.

Other trails have been established primarily for recreational purposes. The paths at Heritage Park and Thompson's Station Park allow area residents to stretch their legs in nature's gym; they offer good views too. The Couchville Lake Trail, a paved all-access loop resembling a running track, is enjoyed by walkers, runners, and those using wheelchairs. Jones Mill Trail, a newer path at Long Hunter State Park, provides hikers and mountain bikers a way to burn some calories.

Then there are greenways, which Nashville and its surrounding communities all seem to be building to enhance the environs. Richland Creek Greenway is a new addition to this edition. Stones River Greenway of Murfreesboro, which cruises alongside the Stones River, connects the town of Murfreesboro with Stones River National Battlefield. The greenway at Shelby Bottoms Nature Park travels beside the Cumberland River not far from downtown Nashville. Cumberland River Bicentennial Trail traces an old railroad bed for miles along bluffs of the lower Cumberland River. And other greenways, such as the Stones River Greenway of Nashville, have been extended.

Finding all these trails became an exciting challenge. And walking them was a joy and a huge learning experience that I am grateful to share with potential readers. Being a native Tennessean, I was familiar with many destinations. Some (such as those at state parks) were obvious, but having written hiking and camping guidebooks about my home state alerted me to more. Being in the hiking world and frequenting outdoors stores helmed by knowledgeable employees helped too. Conveniently, while writing this book, I lived across the street from Warner Parks, Nashville's premier in-town hiking destination. Including those hikes was as easy as walking out the door. My feet also left an extra groove in the Harpeth Woods Trail.

Adding new hikes for this fourth edition was a challenge and a pleasure. I'll admit it—some places were duds that, after I hiked them, had to be eliminated from inclusion. But this book provides the service of doing the literal legwork of finding Nashville's best hikes and providing the details for you, including length, driving directions, scenery, facilities, related activities, and more.

This book will enable you to spend your precious time on the trail rather than finding a trail to get on. I sought to include destinations that had some outstanding feature, whether it was historic appeal, natural beauty, or other activities you can combine with your walk. After hiking the trails included in this book, you too, I hope, will find something special about each one and see what a special place for hiking greater Nashville can be.

60 Hikes by Category

Hike Categories

• mileage • difficulty* • urban • heavily traveled • less busy • kid-friendly

* Difficulty: **E** = easy, **M** = moderate, **D** = difficult

REGION Hike Number/Hike Name	page	mileage	difficulty	urban	heavily traveled	less busy	kid-friendly
NASHVILLE							
1 Bells Bend Loop	14	2.6	E			✓	✓
2 Bryant Grove Trail	18	8.0	M				
3 Couchville Lake Trail	21	2.0	E		✓		✓
4 Ganier Ridge Loop	24	2.4	M	✓		✓	
5 Harpeth Woods Trail	27	2.5	E	✓	✓		
6 Jones Mill Trail	30	3.6	M			✓	
7 MetroCenter Levee Greenway	33	5.8	M	✓	✓		
8 Mill Creek Greenway	36	2.6	E	✓	✓		✓
9 Mossy Ridge Trail	39	4.5	M				
10 Old Hickory Lake Nature Trail	42	1.5	E			✓	✓
11 Peeler Park Hike	45	5.5	M		✓		✓
12 Richland Creek Greenway: McCabe Loop	49	2.8	E–M	✓	✓	✓	
13 Shelby Bottoms Nature Park: East Loop	53	5.2	E		✓	✓	
14 Shelby Bottoms Nature Park: West Loop	57	1.8	E		✓	✓	✓
15 South Radnor Lake Loop	61	2.5	M			✓	
16 Stones River Greenway of Nashville	65	6.0	M	✓	✓	✓	
17 Volunteer–Day Loop	68	4.0	M			✓	
18 Warner Woods Trail	71	2.5	E–M	✓	✓		

REGION Hike Number/Hike Name	page	mileage	difficulty	urban	heavily traveled	less busy	kid-friendly
WEST (including Ashland City, Clarksville, and Dickson)							
19 Confederate Earthworks Walk	76	2.6	M			✓	
20 Cumberland River Bicentennial Trail	79	8.0	M		✓		
21 Dunbar Cave State Natural Park Loop	83	1.8	E			✓	✓
22 Fort Donelson Battlefield Loop	86	3.3	M			✓	
23 Henry Hollow Loop	90	2.1	M			✓	✓
24 Hidden Lake Double Loop	93	1.6	E–M				✓
25 Johnsonville State Historic Park Loop	96	2.6	E–M			✓	
26 Montgomery Bell Northeast Loop	100	6.0	M				
27 Montgomery Bell Southwest Loop	103	6.9	M		✓		
28 Narrows of Harpeth Hike	107	1.8	E		✓		
29 Nathan Bedford Forrest Five-Mile Trail	110	4.9	M			✓	✓
30 Ridgetop Trail at Beaman Park	113	4.2	M				
SOUTHWEST (including Columbia, Fairview, and Franklin)							
31 Devil's Backbone Loop	118	2.7	E–M			✓	✓
32 Gordon House and Ferry Site Walk	121	1.0	E			✓	✓
33 Heritage Park/Thompson's Station Park Hike	125	3.0	M				
34 Lakes of Bowie Loop	128	2.2	E				✓
35 Meriwether Lewis Loop	132	3.5	E–M			✓	
36 Old Trace–Garrison Creek Loop	136	6.3	M	✓		✓	
37 Perimeter Trail	139	5.1	M		✓		
SOUTHEAST (including Brentwood, Murfreesboro, and Smyrna)							
38 Adeline Wilhoite River Trail	144	4.1	M			✓	✓
39 Brenthaven Bikeway Connector	148	2.4	E		✓		
40 Cheeks Bend Bluff View Trail	151	1.8	E				
41 Flat Rock Cedar Glades and Barrens Hike	155	3.4	M				✓
42 Hickory Ridge Trail	159	2.3	E–M				✓
43 Old Mill Trail	163	1.0	E				✓

REGION Hike Number/Hike Name	page	mileage	difficulty	urban	heavily traveled	less busy	kid-friendly
SOUTHEAST (including Brentwood, Murfreesboro, and Smyrna) *(continued)*							
44 Old Stone Fort Loop	166	2.6	M				
45 Short Springs State Natural Area Hike	170	3.2	M				✓
46 Smith Park Hike	174	3.4	M		✓		
47 Stones River Greenway of Murfreesboro	178	6.0	M	✓	✓	✓	
48 Stones River National Battlefield Loop	181	3.3	E				✓
49 Twin Forks Trail	184	1.5	E			✓	
50 Wild Turkey Trail	188	2.5	E			✓	✓
EAST (including Gallatin, Hendersonville, Lebanon, and Mount Juliet)							
51 Bearwaller Gap Hiking Trail	194	11.2	D			✓	
52 Bledsoe Creek State Park Loop	198	3.1	E–M				
53 Cedar Forest Trail	201	2.0	E				✓
54 Collins River Nature Trail	205	3.0	E				✓
55 Eagle Trail	209	1.7	M			✓	
56 Edgar Evins State Park Hike	212	7.9	D	✓			
57 Hidden Springs Trail	215	4.2	E				
58 Sellars Farm State Archaeological Area	218	1.5	E			✓	✓
59 Vesta Glade Trail	222	1.8	E				✓
60 Wilderness Trail	226	12.0	D				

More Hike Categories

• biking • running	• lake • scenic	• wildlife • wildflowers	• historical interest

REGION Hike Number/Hike Name	page	biking	running	lake	scenic	wildlife	wildflowers	historical interest
NASHVILLE								
1 Bells Bend Loop	14		✓			✓		
2 Bryant Grove Trail	18			✓	✓			✓
3 Couchville Lake Trail	21			✓	✓			
4 Ganier Ridge Loop	24				✓		✓	
5 Harpeth Woods Trail	27						✓	✓
6 Jones Mill Trail	30	✓		✓			✓	
7 MetroCenter Levee Greenway	33	✓	✓					
8 Mill Creek Greenway	36	✓	✓					
9 Mossy Ridge Trail	39	✓			✓		✓	✓
10 Old Hickory Lake Nature Trail	42			✓		✓		
11 Peeler Park Hike	45	✓			✓	✓		✓
12 Richland Creek Greenway: McCabe Loop	49	✓	✓					✓
13 Shelby Bottoms Nature Park: East Loop	53	✓	✓		✓			
14 Shelby Bottoms Nature Park: West Loop	57		✓		✓			✓
15 South Radnor Lake Loop	61			✓	✓		✓	
16 Stones River Greenway of Nashville	65	✓	✓		✓			
17 Volunteer–Day Loop	68	✓		✓	✓		✓	
18 Warner Woods Trail	71				✓			
WEST (including Ashland City, Clarksville, and Dickson)								
19 Confederate Earthworks Walk	76							✓
20 Cumberland River Bicentennial Trail	79	✓	✓		✓			
21 Dunbar Cave State Natural Park Loop	83					✓		✓

REGION Hike Number/Hike Name	page	biking	running	lake	scenic	wildlife	wildflowers	historical interest
WEST (including Ashland City, Clarksville, and Dickson) *(continued)*								
22 Fort Donelson Battlefield Loop	86							✓
23 Henry Hollow Loop	90					✓	✓	
24 Hidden Lake Double Loop	93			✓	✓			
25 Johnsonville State Historic Park Loop	96			✓	✓			✓
26 Montgomery Bell Northeast Loop	100	✓					✓	
27 Montgomery Bell Southwest Loop	103						✓	✓
28 Narrows of Harpeth Hike	107				✓			✓
29 Nathan Bedford Forrest Five-Mile Trail	110	✓			✓	✓		
30 Ridgetop Trail at Beaman Park	113	✓				✓		
SOUTHWEST (including Columbia, Fairview, and Franklin)								
31 Devil's Backbone Loop	118				✓		✓	
32 Gordon House and Ferry Site Walk	121							✓
33 Heritage Park/Thompson's Station Park Hike	125				✓			
34 Lakes of Bowie Loop	128			✓		✓		
35 Meriwether Lewis Loop	132				✓		✓	✓
36 Old Trace–Garrison Creek Loop	136							✓
37 Perimeter Trail	139	✓						
SOUTHEAST (including Brentwood, Murfreesboro, and Smyrna)								
38 Adeline Wilhoite River Trail	144	✓			✓	✓	✓	✓
39 Brenthaven Bikeway Connector	148		✓					
40 Cheeks Bend Bluff View Trail	151				✓			
41 Flat Rock Cedar Glades and Barrens Hike	155	✓			✓		✓	
42 Hickory Ridge Trail	159				✓			✓

REGION Hike Number/Hike Name	page	biking	running	lake	scenic	wildlife	wildflowers	historical interest
SOUTHEAST (including Brentwood, Murfreesboro, and Smyrna) *(continued)*								
43 Old Mill Trail	163							✓
44 Old Stone Fort Loop	166				✓		✓	✓
45 Short Springs State Natural Area Hike	170				✓		✓	
46 Smith Park Hike	174	✓	✓				✓	✓
47 Stones River Greenway of Murfreesboro	178	✓	✓					✓
48 Stones River National Battlefield Loop	181	✓						✓
49 Twin Forks Trail	184			✓	✓	✓		
50 Wild Turkey Trail	188					✓		
EAST (including Gallatin, Hendersonville, Lebanon, and Mount Juliet)								
51 Bearwaller Gap Hiking Trail	194			✓	✓	✓	✓	
52 Bledsoe Creek State Park Loop	198			✓		✓		
53 Cedar Forest Trail	201				✓			
54 Collins River Nature Trail	205	✓			✓	✓		
55 Eagle Trail	209				✓		✓	
56 Edgar Evins State Park Hike	212			✓	✓			✓
57 Hidden Springs Trail	215	✓				✓		
58 Sellars Farm State Archaeological Area	218		✓		✓			✓
59 Vesta Glade Trail	222				✓		✓	
60 Wilderness Trail	226			✓	✓	✓		

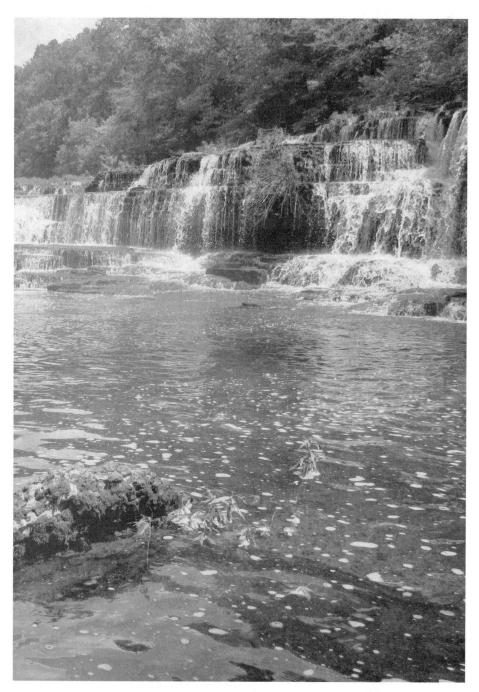

One of the many waterfalls found on the Old Stone Fort Loop (see page 166)

Introduction

WELCOME TO *60 Hikes Within 60 Miles: Nashville!* If you're new to hiking, or even if you're a seasoned trailsmith, take a few minutes to read the following introduction. We'll explain how this book is organized and how to get the best use of it.

How to Use This Guidebook

THE OVERVIEW MAP, MAP KEY, AND MAP LEGEND

Use the overview map on the inside front cover to assess the general location of each hike's primary trailhead. Each hike's number appears on the overview map, on the map key facing the overview map, and in the table of contents. Flipping through the book, you will easily locate a hike's full profile by watching for the hike number at the top of each page. The book is organized by region, as indicated in the table of contents. A map legend that details the symbols found on the trail maps can be found on the inside back cover.

REGIONAL MAPS

The book is divided into regions, and prefacing each regional section is an overview map of that region. The regional map provides more detail than the overview map does, bringing you closer to the hike.

HIKE PROFILES

Each hike profile contains seven key items: a brief description of the trail, a Key At-a-Glance Information box, GPS coordinates, directions to the trailhead, a trail map, a hike description, and information on nearby activities when applicable. Combined, the maps and information provide a clear method to assess each trail from the comfort of your favorite reading chair.

IN BRIEF

Think of this section as a taste of the trail, a snapshot focused on the historical landmarks, beautiful vistas, and other sights you may encounter on the trail.

KEY AT-A-GLANCE INFORMATION

The information boxes give you a quick idea of the specifics of each hike. Twelve basic elements are covered.

DISTANCE & CONFIGURATION Options are often provided to shorten or extend the hikes, but the mileage corresponds to the described hike. Consult the hike description to decide how to customize the hike for your ability or time constraints. This element also describes what the trail might look like from overhead. Trails can be loops, out-and-backs (that is, along the same route), figure eights, or balloons. Sometimes the descriptions might surprise you.

DIFFICULTY   The degree of effort an average hiker should expect on a given hike. For simplicity, difficulty is described as easy, moderate, or difficult.

SCENERY   A summary of the overall environs of the hike and what to expect in terms of plant life, wildlife, streams, and historic buildings.

EXPOSURE   A quick check of how much sun you can expect on your shoulders during the hike. Descriptors used are self-explanatory and include terms such as *shady, exposed,* and *sunny.*

TRAFFIC   Indicates how busy the trail might be on an average day and if you might be able to find solitude out there. Trail traffic, of course, varies from day to day and season to season.

TRAIL SURFACE   Indicates whether the trail is paved, rocky, smooth dirt, or a mixture of elements.

HIKING TIME   How long it took the author to hike the trail. Estimated times are based on an average pace of 2 to 3 miles per hour, adjusted for the ease or difficulty of the hike's terrain. Hikes with wide-ranging time estimates describe trail networks with hiking options of varying lengths. Keep in mind that if you're a birder, wildflower lover, amateur geologist, or a doze-on-rocks type like the author, hike times will be quite a bit longer.

ACCESS   Notes time of day when hike route is open, days when it is closed, and when permits or fees are needed to access the trail.

PETS   Notes if pets are allowed on the trail and, if so, whether a leash is required.

MAPS   Which map is the best, or easiest to read (in the author's opinion) for this hike, and where to get it.

FACILITIES   What to expect in terms of restrooms, phones, water, and other niceties available at the trailhead or nearby.

CONTACT   Phone numbers and websites, where applicable, for up-to-date information on trail conditions.

LOCATION   The city in which the trail is located.

COMMENTS   Provides you with those extra details that don't fit into any of the above categories. Here you'll find information on trail hiking options and facts such as whether or not to expect a lifeguard at a nearby swimming beach.

DESCRIPTION

The trail description is the heart of each hike. Here, the author provides a summary of the trail's essence, as well as a highlight of any special traits the hike offers. Ultimately, the hike description will help you choose which hikes are best for you.

NEARBY ACTIVITIES

Not every hike will have this listing. For those that do, look here for information on nearby sights of interest.

DIRECTIONS

Used with the locator map, the directions will help you locate each trailhead. When possible, directions to hikes begin from the nearest interstate exit off highways leading from Nashville. Directions to trails far from expressways start from nearby towns or major highway intersections.

TRAIL MAPS

Each hike contains a detailed map that shows the trailhead, the route, significant features, facilities, and topographic landmarks such as creeks, overlooks, and peaks. Each trailhead's GPS coordinates are included with each profile.

GPS TRAILHEAD COORDINATES

In addition to highly specific trail outlines, this book also includes the latitude (north) and longitude (west) coordinates for each trailhead. The latitude–longitude grid system is likely quite familiar to you, but here's a refresher, pertinent to visualizing the coordinates.

Imaginary lines of latitude—called parallels and approximately 69 miles apart from each other—run horizontally around the globe. Each parallel is indicated by degrees from the equator (established to be 0°): up to 90°N at the North Pole and down to 90°S at the South Pole.

Imaginary lines of longitude—called meridians—run perpendicular to lines of latitude and are likewise indicated by degrees. Starting from 0° at the Prime Meridian in Greenwich, England, they continue to the east and west until they meet 180° later at the International Date Line in the Pacific Ocean. At the equator, longitude lines also are approximately 69 miles apart, but that distance narrows as the meridians converge toward the North and South Poles.

Topographic maps show latitude–longitude. The survey datum used to arrive at the coordinates in this book is WGS84 (versus NAD27 or WGS83). For readers who own a GPS unit, whether a handheld device, on their smartphone, or onboard a vehicle, the latitude–longitude coordinates provided with each hike may be entered into the GPS unit. Just make sure your GPS unit is set to navigate using WGS84 datum. Now you can navigate directly to the trailhead.

In this book, latitude and longitude are expressed in degree–decimal minute format. For example, the coordinates for Hike 1, Bells Bend Loop (page 14), are as follows: N36° 9.367'   W86° 55.570'.

Most trailheads, which begin in parking areas, can be reached by car, but some hikes still require a short walk to reach the trailhead from a parking area. In those cases a hand-held unit is necessary to continue the GPS navigation process. That said, however, readers can easily access all trailheads in this book by using the directions given, the overview map, and the trail map, which shows at least one major road leading into the area. But for those who enjoy using the latest GPS technology to navigate, the necessary data has been provided. For more on GPS technology, visit **usgs.gov.**

TOPO MAPS

The maps in this book have been produced with great care. When used with the route directions in each profile, the maps are sufficient to direct you to the trail and guide you on it. However, you will find superior detail and valuable information in the United States Geological Survey's (USGS) 7.5-minute series topographic maps.

Topo maps are available online in many locations. At **mytopo.com**, for example, you can view and print topos of the entire Unites States free of charge. Online services, such as **trails.com**, charge annual fees for additional features such as shaded relief, which makes the topography stand out more. If you expect to print out many topo maps each year, it might be worth paying for shaded-relief topo maps. The downside to USGS topos is that most of them are outdated, having been created 20–30 years ago. But they still provide excellent topographic detail. Of course, **Google Earth** (**earth.google.com**) does away with topo maps and their inaccuracies—replacing them with satellite imagery and its inaccuracies. Regardless, what one lacks, the other augments. Google Earth is an excellent tool whether you have difficulty with topos or not.

If you're new to hiking, you might be wondering, "What's a topographic map?" In short, a topo indicates not only linear distance but elevation as well, using contour lines. Contour lines spread across the map like dozens of intricate spider webs. Each line represents a particular elevation, and at the base of each topo, a contour's interval designation is given. If the contour interval is 20 feet, then the distance between each contour line is 20 feet. Follow five contour lines up on the same map, and the elevation has increased by 100 feet.

Let's assume that the 7.5-minute series topo reads "Contour Interval 40 feet," that the short trail we'll be hiking is 2 inches in length on the map, and that it crosses five contour lines from beginning to end. What do we know? Well, because the linear scale of this series is 2,000 feet to the inch (roughly 2.75 inches representing 1 mile), we know our trail is approximately 0.8 mile long (2 inches equals 2,000 feet). But we also know we'll be climbing or descending 200 vertical feet (five contour lines are 40 feet each) over that

AVERAGE TEMPERATURE BY MONTH FOR NASHVILLE, TENNESSEE						
	JAN	FEB	MAR	APR	MAY	JUN
Min	21°F	27°F	36°F	47°F	57°F	66°F
Max	38°F	44°F	55°F	67°F	77°F	85°F
Mean	30°F	35°F	46°F	57°F	67°F	76°F
	JUL	AUG	SEP	OCT	NOV	DEC
Min	71°F	69°F	60°F	48°F	37°F	26°F
Max	90°F	88°F	80°F	68°F	54°F	42°F
Mean	80°F	78°F	70°F	56°F	45°F	34°F

distance. And the elevation designations written on occasional contour lines will tell us if we're heading up or down.

In addition to the outdoor shops listed in the Appendix, you'll find topos at major universities and some public libraries, where you might try photocopying the ones you need to avoid the cost of buying them. But if you want your own and can't find them locally, visit **nationalmap.gov** or **store.usgs.gov.**

Weather

While any time is fine for hiking in the Nashville area, spring and fall are most folks' favorite seasons. The first warm breath of spring brings wildflowers, and seasonal rains bring the streams to life—waterfalls and cascades are everywhere in April and May. October brings spectacular fall colors, along with crisp, cool days free of bugs and humidity.

Winter is my favorite time to hike: no bugs, no heat or humidity, and best of all, no foliage. Vistas obscured by greenery in the warm months open up in winter, and when it's really cold, the streams, waterfalls, and seeps create incredible ice formations. Summer, with its heat and humidity, is a tough time to hike around Nashville. Get out early in the morning, or try something really unique—choose a park open after sunset and hike by the light of the full moon.

Water

How much is enough? Well, one simple physiological fact should convince you to err on the side of excess when deciding how much water to pack: A hiker working hard in 90° heat needs approximately 10 quarts of fluid per day. That's 2.5 gallons—12 large water bottles or 16 small ones. In other words, pack one or two bottles even for short hikes.

Some hikers and backpackers hit the trail prepared to purify water found along the route. This method, while less dangerous than drinking untreated water, comes with risks. Purifiers with ceramic filters are the safest. Many hikers pack the slightly distasteful

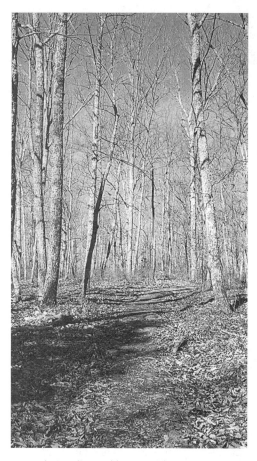

Lonely Devil's Backbone trail among winter hardwoods (see page 118)

tetraglycine-hydroperiodide tablets (sold under the names Potable Aqua, Coughlan's, etc.) to debug water.

Probably the most common waterborne "bug" that hikers face is *Giardia,* which may not hit until one to four weeks after ingestion. It will have you living in the bathroom, passing noxious rotten-egg gas, vomiting, and shivering with chills. Other parasites to worry about include *E. coli* and *Cryptosporidium,* both of which are harder to kill than *Giardia.*

For most people, the pleasures of hiking make carrying water a relatively minor price to pay to remain healthy. If you are tempted to drink "found" water, do so only if you understand the risks involved. Better yet, hydrate prior to your hike, carry (and drink) 6 ounces of water for every mile you plan to hike, and hydrate again after the hike.

Clothing

There is a wide variety of clothing from which to choose. Basically, use common sense and be prepared for anything. If all you have are cotton clothes when a sudden rainstorm comes along, you'll be miserable, especially in cooler weather. It's a good idea to carry a light wool sweater or some type of synthetic apparel (polypropylene, Capilene, Thermax, and so on) as well as a hat.

Be aware of the weather forecast and its tendency to be wrong. Always carry raingear. Thunderstorms can come on suddenly in the summer. Keep in mind that rainy days are as much a part of nature as those idyllic ones you desire. Besides, rainy days really cut down on the crowds. With appropriate raingear, a normally crowded trail can be a wonderful place of solitude. Do, however, remain aware of the dangers of lightning strikes.

Footwear is another concern. Though tennis shoes may be appropriate for paved areas, some trails are rocky and rough; tennis shoes may not offer enough support. Waterproofed or not, boots should be your footwear of choice. Sport sandals are more popular than ever, but these leave much of your foot exposed, making you vulnerable to hazardous plants, thorns, or the occasional piece of glass.

The 10 Essentials

One of the first rules of hiking is to be prepared for anything. The simplest way to be prepared is to carry the "10 Essentials," listed below. In addition to carrying them, you need to know how to use them, especially navigation items. Always consider worst-case scenarios like getting lost, hiking back in the dark, having broken gear (for example, a broken hip strap on your pack or a plugged water filter), twisting an ankle, or a brutal thunderstorm. The items listed below don't cost a lot of money, don't take up much room in a pack, and don't weigh much, but they might just save your life.

- ➢ *Water:* durable bottles and water treatment like iodine or a filter
- ➢ *Maps:* preferably a topographic map and a trail map that includes a route description
- ➢ *Compass:* a high-quality compass
- ➢ *First-aid kit:* a good-quality kit, including first-aid instructions
- ➢ *Knife:* a multitool device with pliers
- ➢ *Light:* flashlight or headlamp with extra bulbs and batteries
- ➢ *Fire:* windproof matches or a lighter and fire starter
- ➢ *Extra food:* You should always have food in your pack when you've finished hiking.
- ➢ *Extra clothes:* rain protection, warm layers, gloves, warm hat
- ➢ *Sun protection:* sunglasses, lip balm, sunblock, sun hat

First-Aid Kit

A typical first-aid kit may contain more items than you might think necessary. The list of supplies here covers just the basics. Prepackaged kits in waterproof bags (Atwater Carey and Adventure Medical make a variety of kits) are also available. Even though quite a few items are listed here, they pack down into a small space:

- ➢ Ace bandages or Spenco joint wraps
- ➢ Antibiotic ointment *(Neosporin or the generic equivalent)*
- ➢ Aspirin or acetaminophen
- ➢ Band-Aids
- ➢ Benadryl or the generic equivalent—diphenhydramine *(an antihistamine, in case of allergic reactions)*
- ➢ Butterfly-closure bandages

➢ Epinephrine in a prefilled syringe *(for those known to have severe allergic reactions to such things as bee stings)*

➢ Gauze (one roll)

➢ Gauze compress pads *(a half dozen 4-inch by 4-inch)*

➢ Hydrogen peroxide or iodine

➢ Insect repellent

➢ Matches or pocket lighter

➢ Moleskin/Spenco "Second Skin"

➢ Snakebite kit

➢ Sunscreen

➢ Water-purification tablets or water filter *(on longer hikes)*

➢ Whistle (more effective in signaling rescuers than your voice)

Pack the items in a waterproof bag such as a zip-top bag. You will also want to include a snack for hikes longer than a couple of miles. A bag full of GORP (good ol' raisins and peanuts) will kick up your energy level fast.

Hiking with Children

No one is too young for a hike in the outdoors. Be mindful, though. Flat, short, and shaded trails are best with an infant. Toddlers who have not quite mastered walking can still tag along, riding on an adult's back in a child carrier. Use common sense to judge a child's capacity to hike a particular trail, and always assume that the child will tire quickly and need to be carried.

When packing for the hike, remember the child's needs as well as your own. Make sure children are adequately clothed for the weather, have proper shoes, and are protected from the sun with sunscreen. Kids dehydrate quickly, so make sure you have plenty of fluid for everyone. To assist an adult with determining which trails are suitable for youngsters, a list of hike recommendations for children is provided on pages xii–xiv.

General Safety

No doubt, potentially dangerous situations can occur outdoors, but as long as you use sound judgment and prepare yourself before hitting the trail, you'll be safer in the woods than in most urban areas of the country. It is better to look at a backcountry hike as a fascinating chance to discover the unknown rather than a chance for potential disaster. Here are a few tips to make your trip safer and easier.

➢ *Always carry food and water* whether you are planning to go overnight or not. Food will give you energy, help keep you warm, and sustain you in an emergency situation until help arrives. You never know if you will have a stream nearby when you become thirsty. Bring potable water or treat water before drinking it from a stream. Boil or filter all found water before drinking it.

➤ *Stay on designated trails*. Most hikers get lost when they leave the path. Even on the most clearly marked trails, there is usually a point where you have to stop and consider which direction to head. If you become disoriented, don't panic. As soon as you think you may be off track, stop, assess your current direction, and then retrace your steps back to the point where you went awry. Using map, compass, and this book, and keeping in mind what you have passed thus far, reorient yourself and trust your judgment on which way to continue. If you become absolutely unsure of how to continue, return to your vehicle the way you came in. Should you become completely lost and have no idea how to return to the trailhead, remaining in place along the trail and waiting for help is most often the best option for adults and always the best option for children.

➤ *Be especially careful when crossing streams*. Whether you are fording the stream or crossing on a log, make every step count. If you have any doubt about maintaining your balance on a foot log, go ahead and ford the stream instead. When fording a stream, use a trekking pole or stout stick for balance, and face upstream as you cross. If a stream seems too deep to ford, turn back. Whatever is on the other side is not worth risking your life.

➤ *Be careful at overlooks*. While these areas may provide spectacular views, they are potentially hazardous. Stay back from the edge of outcrops, and be absolutely sure of your footing; a misstep can mean a nasty or possibly fatal fall.

➤ *Standing dead trees and storm-damaged living trees can pose a real hazard* to hikers and tent campers. These trees may have loose or broken limbs that could fall at any time. When choosing a spot to rest or a backcountry campsite, look up.

➤ *Know the symptoms of hypothermia*. Shivering and forgetfulness are the two most common indicators of this insipid killer. Hypothermia can occur at any elevation, even in the summer, especially when the hiker is wearing lightweight cotton clothing. If symptoms arise, get the victim shelter, hot liquids, and dry clothes or a dry sleeping bag.

➤ *Take along your brain*. A cool, calculating mind is the single most important piece of equipment you'll ever need on the trail. Think before you act. Watch your step. Plan ahead. Avoiding accidents before they happen is the best recipe for a rewarding and relaxing hike.

Animal and Plant Hazards

TICKS

Ticks like to hang out in the brush that grows along trails. Hot summer months seem to explode their numbers, but you should be tick-aware during all months of the year. Ticks, which are arthropods and not insects, need a host to feast on in order to reproduce. The ticks that light onto you while you hike will be very small, sometimes so tiny that you won't be able to spot them. Both of the primary varieties, deer ticks and dog ticks, need a few hours of actual attachment before they can transmit any disease they may harbor.

Ticks may settle in shoes, socks, and hats and may take several hours to actually latch on. The best strategy is to visually check every half hour or so while hiking, do a thorough check before you get in the car, and then, when you take a posthike shower, do an even more thorough check of your entire body. Ticks that haven't attached are easily removed but not easily killed. If you pick off a tick in the woods, just toss it aside. If you find one on your body at home, dispatch it and then send it down the toilet. For ticks that have embedded, removal with tweezers is best.

SNAKES

Tennessee is home to 32 types of snakes, 4 of which are venomous. Consider yourself lucky if you see a snake, acknowledging that snakes are part of the great Middle Tennessee ecosystem. Refrain from messing with them. All of the Volunteer State's venomous snakes have a vertical, elliptical-shaped pupil and are generally heavy bodied. The timber rattler and copperhead are found throughout Middle Tennessee. The two others, cottonmouth and pygmy rattler, can be found west of the Nashville Basin. You might spend a few minutes studying snakes before heading into the woods, but a good rule of thumb is to give whatever animal you encounter a wide berth and leave it alone.

POISON IVY, POISON OAK, AND POISON SUMAC

Recognizing poison ivy, oak, and sumac and avoiding contact with them is the most effective way to prevent the painful, itchy rashes associated with these plants. Poison ivy ranges from a thick tree-hugging vine to a shaded ground cover, 3 leaflets to a leaf; poison oak occurs as either a vine or a shrub, with 3 leaflets as well; and poison sumac flourishes in swampland, each leaf containing 7–13 leaflets. Urushiol, the oil in the sap of these plants, is responsible for the rash. Usually within 12 to 14 hours of exposure (but sometimes much later), raised lines and/or blisters will appear, accompanied by a terrible itch. Refrain from scratching because bacteria under fingernails can cause infection and you will spread the rash to other parts of your body. Wash and dry the rash thoroughly, applying a calamine lotion or other product to help dry the rash. If itching or blistering is severe, seek medical attention. Remember that oil-contaminated clothes, pets, or hiking gear can easily cause an irritating rash on you or someone else, so wash not only any exposed parts of your body but also clothes, gear, and pets.

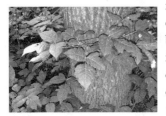

poison ivy

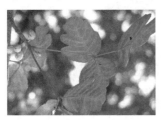

poison oak

MOSQUITOES

Though it's very rare, individuals can become infected with the West Nile virus by being bitten by an infected mosquito. Culex mosquitoes, the primary varieties that can transmit West Nile virus to humans, thrive in urban rather than natural areas. They lay their eggs in stagnant water and can breed in any standing water that remains for more than five days. Most people infected with West Nile virus have no symptoms of illness, but some may become ill, usually 3–15 days after being bitten.

Anytime you expect mosquitoes to be buzzing around, you may want to wear protective clothing such as long sleeves, long pants, and socks. Loose-fitting, light-colored clothing is best. Spray clothing with insect repellent. Remember to follow the instructions on the repellent and to take extra care with children.

The Business Hiker

Whether you're in the Nashville area on business as a resident or an out-of-towner, the hikes in this book afford the perfect opportunity to make a quick getaway from the demands of commerce. Some of the hikes classified as urban are located close to office areas and are easily accessible from downtown areas.

Instead of buying a burger down the street, pack a lunch and head for a nearby trail to take a relaxing break from the office or that tiresome convention. Or plan ahead and take along a small group of your business comrades. A well-planned half-day getaway is the perfect complement to a business stay in Nashville or any of the other close-in communities in the metropolitan area.

Trail Etiquette

Whether you're on a city, county, state, or national park trail, always remember that great care and resources (from nature as well as from your tax dollars) have gone into creating these trails. Treat the trail, wildlife, and fellow hikers with respect.

Here are a few general ideas to keep in mind while on the trail:

1. Hike on open trails only. Respect trail and road closures (ask if you're not sure), avoid trespassing on private land, and obtain any required permits or authorization. Leave gates as you found them or as marked.

2. Leave no trace of your visit other than footprints. Be sensitive to the land beneath your feet. This also means staying on the trail and not creating any new trails. Be sure to pack out what you pack in. No one likes to see trash that someone else has left behind.

3. Never spook animals; give them extra room and time to adjust to you.

4. Plan ahead. Know your equipment, your ability, and the area in which you are hiking—and prepare accordingly. Be self-sufficient at all times; carry necessary supplies for changes in weather or other conditions. A well-executed trip is a satisfaction to you and not a burden or offense to others.

5. Be courteous to other hikers, bikers, and all people you meet while hiking.

NASHVILLE

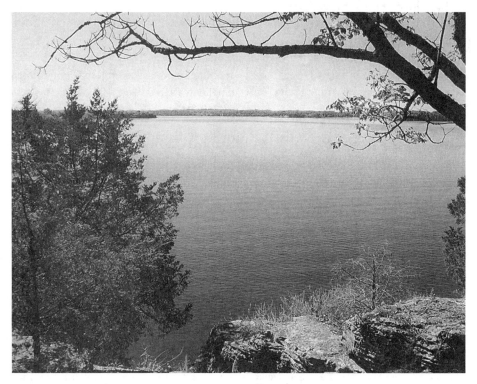

Soak in a view of J. Percy Priest Lake along the Volunteer–Day Loop (see page 68).

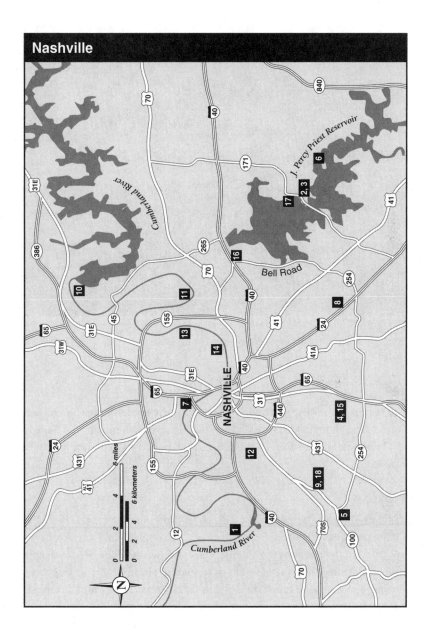

Nashville

1 Bells Bend Loop

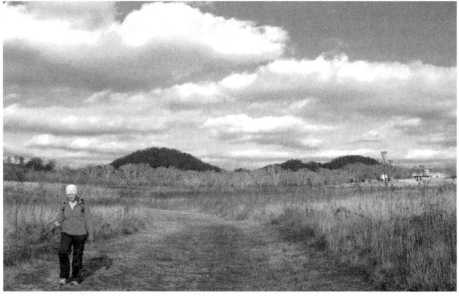

photographed by Jody Stickle

A hiker braves a cold but sunny day.

In Brief

Bells Bend Park is the setting for this loop hike along the banks of the Cumberland River. It travels through rolling fields and alongside the big river, where you can enjoy vistas of hills and bluffs before returning to the trailhead. Opened in 2007, the park also has a nature center.

Description

Talk about turning bad into good. The city of Nashville purchased the Bells Bend area back in 1989 for use as a landfill. Luckily, former mayor Bill Purcell had other ideas for this scenic tract on the banks of the Cumberland, and two decades later we have a scenic park with hiking trails. Now the 800-plus-acre tract of land is a mix of woods and open areas set along a picturesque arc of land west of downtown. The former farmland still has wooded fence lines, old farm ponds, and even a barn. Nonetheless, the park is a green oasis, and its natural amenities are being enhanced. Keep in mind that shade is limited, so this may not be a desirable summertime trek.

Leave the parking area and trailhead and immediately cross an intermittent creek on an iron bridge. The gravel track cuts across a field and then two lines of trees to reach a

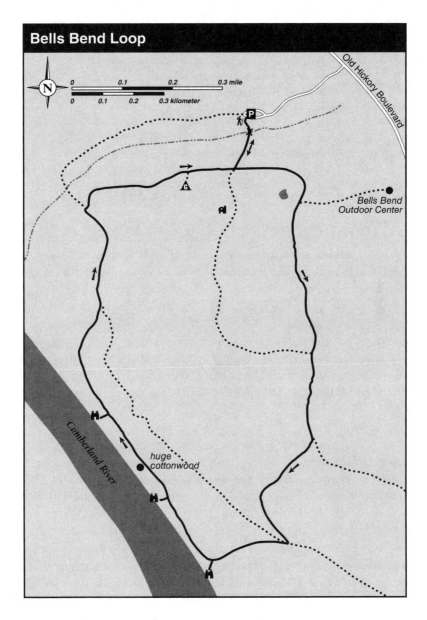

Bells Bend Loop

trail junction at 0.1 mile. Here, extremely wide grassy tracks branch to the left and right, while the gravel trail continues straight. Head left (east). Bells Bend Outdoor Center stands atop a hill in the distance. This is easily the widest trail in this entire guidebook, perhaps extending 12 feet wide. You don't quite make the nature center, as the trail curves south and reaches a junction at 0.3 mile. Continue straight as another superwide trail leads left to the nature center. Note the trailside pond.

DISTANCE AND CONFIGURATION: 2.6-mile loop	**ACCESS:** No fees or permits required
DIFFICULTY: Easy	**PETS:** On leash only
SCENERY: Open fields, Cumberland River floodplain, bluffs	**MAPS:** USGS *Scottsboro;* at **tinyurl.com/bellsbendmap**
EXPOSURE: Mostly sunny	**FACILITIES:** Nature center near trail-head, variable hours
TRAFFIC: Moderate on weekends	
TRAIL SURFACE: Gravel, grass, a little asphalt	**CONTACT:** 615-862-4187; **tinyurl.com/bellsbendpark**
HIKING TIME: 1.3 hours	**LOCATION:** Nashville

The loop continues meandering south through fields of grass and briars. Lines of trees delineate the fields, while the hills and bluffs of the Cumberland River rise in the distance. The open landscape lies bare the contours of the land. At 0.6 mile, a shortcut trail leads right, toward the trailhead. Here you'll reach the highest point of the hike, with views stretching out to the back and beyond. One thing you'll note is the prevalence of cell towers, radio towers, and other communication towers that reflect our modern life. Pass through another line of trees at 0.7 mile and begin descending to another junction. Here, a combination of trails and old farm roads make a mini loop of their own. This hike stays right, aiming for the Cumberland River. Cedars and hackberry trees form a treeline to your right.

At 1.1 miles, intersect the aforementioned mini loop. Keep shooting for the big water, as yet another trail runs the margin between the floodplain and the hills. You are now in the river floodplain, which comprises 30% of this park. Soon you'll come to the river, where a screen of cane and trees grows along the banks. A spur trail leads down to a view of the river, and a mud trail descends to the water's edge. The mud trail was created by dogs—and a few humans—who just can't fight the lure of the water. Travel northwest along the mighty Cumberland, which flows strongly to meet the Ohio River. At 1.4 miles, pass another river clearing. The bluffs across the river rise nearly 400 feet from the water. Most of the trees along the river's edge are small, but you do pass a huge cottonwood at 1.5 miles. It looks old enough to have seen an American Indian float by in a dugout canoe.

Climb away from the river and pass the other end of the trail that runs along the floodplain at 1.9 miles. Continue heading toward the trailhead, passing a trail that leads left to cross the stream passing near the trailhead. The main trail heads east and meets the park's group camp at 2.4 miles. Keep straight here to reach another junction and the loop's end at 2.5 miles. Turn left here, backtracking to the trailhead, and complete your hike at 2.6 miles. Just think, this could've been a landfill.

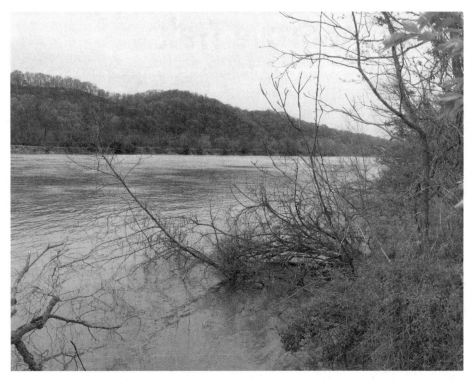

The mighty Cumberland River as it flows past Bells Bend

Nearby Activities

Bells Bend Outdoor Center is located at the park. It is currently open Tuesday–Friday, noon–4 p.m., and Saturday, 9 a.m.–4 p.m. For more information, visit **tinyurl.com /bellsbendnc**.

GPS TRAILHEAD COORDINATES
N36° 9.367' W86° 55.570'

From Exit 24 on TN 155/Briley Parkway, northwest of downtown, take TN 12 North/ Ashland City Highway 2.7 miles west to Old Hickory Boulevard. Turn left onto Old Hickory Boulevard and follow it 4.2 miles to the right turn into Bells Bend Park. Follow this road to dead-end at the trailhead in 0.1 mile.

2 Bryant Grove Trail

In Brief

This out-and-back hike cruises through Long Hunter State Park, along the pretty shoreline of J. Percy Priest Lake. The walking is easy, but the total distance—if you make the entire hike—is 8 miles. You may see wading birds and waterfowl in season.

Description

Bryant Grove Trail is your best bet for solitude at Long Hunter State Park. The path starts in the busy Couchville Lake Day Use Area and then heads east into solitude along the shore of J. Percy Priest Lake. The wide trail bed is easy to follow as it meanders through cedar thickets, oak–hickory forests, and cedar glades to swing around the Bryant Creek embayment. It ends at Bryant Grove Recreation Area, where picnic tables and a swim beach await. Be aware—this is not a loop trail. The 4 miles out, though easy with no real hills, require 4 miles back to the trailhead, unless you leave another car at Bryant Grove Recreation Area, which is a 7-mile drive from the Couchville Lake Day Use Area.

Start the Bryant Grove Trail by leaving the Couchville Lake Day Use Area and tracing the gravel path into cedar woods. Couchville Lake and Couchville Lake Trail are off to your left. Shortly pick up the old bed of O'Neals Ford Road. You'll notice that the canopy gives way overhead and J. Percy Priest Lake is off to your right. In the winter, when the lake pool is drawn down, you can see the rockiness of the lake bed. In the woods to your left, vast amounts of stone protrude above what little soil exists in this karst topography, where the limestone lies at or near the land surface. Pockets of rich soil do occur here, which is usually indicated by the presence of oak–hickory forests. In less-rich soil, cedars dominate. The poorest soils or the areas with the least amount of dirt (and most exposed rock) harbor cedar glades.

Wooden posts mark the trail's progression at 0.5-mile increments. Climb a small hill just past the 0.5-mile post; then make a hard left, leaving the lake and roadbed. A sign here reads TRAIL DOES NOT LOOP, reminding hikers that every step they hike out, they will have to hike back. Look for a crumbling, old stone wall in the woods off to your right. You may also see wooden posts supporting barbed wire. These lands, too rocky for large-scale agriculture, were used for grazing in prepark days.

Look left at the 1-mile post for a cedar glade. Bryant Grove Trail veers right here and picks up another woods road to enter terrain that slopes toward the lake. Begin curving around the Bryant Creek embayment and arrive near the shore before reaching a signboard and kiosk indicating the halfway point of the trail at 2 miles. Just past the kiosk, the Bryant Grove Trail crosses an unnamed wet-weather stream. Rocks have been placed across the crossing, enabling hikers to keep their feet dry even after winter rains, when this stream is likely to be running. In fall, it may be nearly dry.

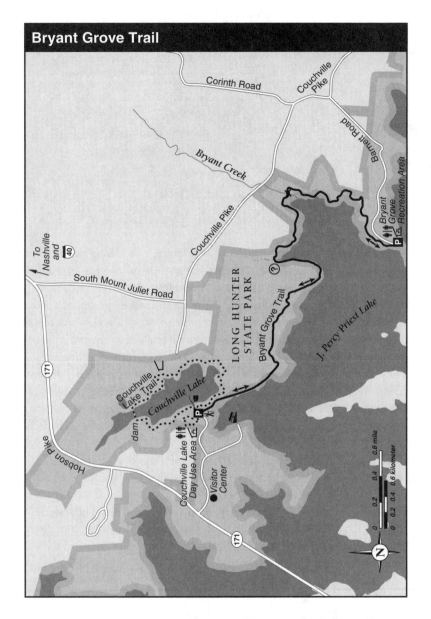

Bryant Grove Trail

Keep curving around the cove, and soon you'll be traveling directly along the shore-line. Views stretch far onto J. Percy Priest Lake, and birds, such as herons, may be wading in the embayment. Bryant Grove Trail continues along the shore to reach Bryant Creek at mile 2.8; a wooden bridge with handrails allows dry passage. Turn downstream along Bryant Creek, where you can see the stream flow into the lake. Look across the creek at a stone wall along the creek bank that kept Bryant Creek in check in days gone by. (The rich soil along the creek may have been used for a family's vegetable garden.) Another stone wall is visible across the water above the creek bank.

DISTANCE AND CONFIGURATION: 8-mile out-and-back	**PETS:** Not allowed on this trail
DIFFICULTY: Moderate	**MAPS:** USGS *La Vergne*; at **tinyurl.com/longhuntermap**
SCENERY: Lake, cedar thickets, hardwood forest, cedar glades	**FACILITIES:** Restrooms, water at trailhead
EXPOSURE: More shady than sunny	**CONTACT:** 615-885-2422; **tnstateparks**
TRAFFIC: Moderate	**.com/parks/about/long-hunter**
TRAIL SURFACE: Gravel, rocks, dirt	**LOCATION:** Hermitage
HIKING TIME: 4 hours	**COMMENTS:** You can start the trail on either end.
ACCESS: No fees or permits required	

Pass a small feeder stream on a boardwalk, and look left for a larger glade growing up in young, bushy cedars. Bryant Grove Trail then enters a dense cedar thicket that forms a dark, cool pocket no matter the time of year. Emerge from the thicket and enter a gravelly glade at mile 3.4. The openness of the sky at this point will make you squint. This area contains the poorest of poor soil from a farmer's perspective but is rare, rich land to a botanist. *Land* isn't even the right word for this area because it really is an extensive flat of broken limestone rock. In the cracks and crevices are wildflowers and rare plants that grow only in these glades, making Middle Tennessee home to a unique American environment.

Drift among more open glades, and then ascend through a rocky hardwood forest to reach Bryant Grove Recreation Area at 4 miles. Here you'll find picnic tables, grills, a restroom, a boat launch, and a swim beach. If you haven't left a shuttle car here, it is time to backtrack to Couchville Lake Day Use Area.

Early to late spring is the best time to view wildflowers along this trail. However, keep in mind that heavy winter and spring rains tend to wash over the trail, rendering it impassable across Bryant Creek (despite the bridge) and over the O'Neals Ford roadbed from the Couchville Lake side. Call ahead if you are concerned about high water.

Nearby Activities

The park has a fishing pier and rents canoes and small johnboats. No gas motors are allowed, which makes for a peaceful experience.

GPS TRAILHEAD COORDINATES
N36° 5.583' W86° 32.625'

From Exit 226 on I-40, east of downtown Nashville, take TN 171 South/South Mount Juliet Road 4.2 miles south. Veer right at the split, as TN 171 becomes Hobson Pike. Continue 2.4 miles, turning left into the Couchville Lake Day Use Area. Continue 0.4 mile and turn left into Area Two. Soon reach the parking area and trailhead. The trail starts near the playground on the right side of the parking area as you enter it.

3 Couchville Lake Trail

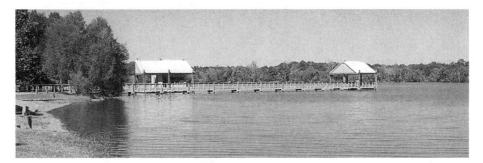

A pier stretches into Couchville Lake

In Brief

This easy trail circles Couchville Lake, which lies adjacent to J. Percy Priest Lake at Long Hunter State Park. The popular paved path winds through woods and has many side trails leading to small piers on the lake's edge. Tree- and plant-identification signs enhance the experience. And a 300-foot bridge that spans the lake offers panoramic views. You may also see wildlife on the lake and in the woods on quiet mornings.

Description

Long Hunter State Park did a fine job laying out this trail. The 8-foot-wide, nearly level path makes up in beauty what it lacks in challenge. But that is the very point of this trail—to be accessible for folks with disabilities as well as for the average walker. Those developing Long Hunter State Park actually had no idea what a good recreation destination Couchville Lake would become because they had no idea Couchville Lake would ever exist. Before the Stones River was dammed and J. Percy Priest Lake was formed, the area that would later become Couchville Lake was just a big depression. When J. Percy Priest Lake filled, water seeped from the impoundment through underground passages to fill the depression, forming Couchville Lake. And this relationship between Percy Priest and Couchville continues: When J. Percy Priest Lake goes up or down, so goes Couchville Lake.

Leave the parking area and head toward the fishing pier and canoes stored at the lake's edge. Here you'll turn right onto the trail, which is marked in 0.5-mile increments. Couchville Lake will be to your left. Leave the open lakeshore to find a woodland area of cedar, walnut, and oak. Soon you'll see the first of many interpretive signs, which inform hikers about the trees and plants around them.

At 0.2 mile, the level path circles to the left and passes the first of several small lakeside observation piers. Bird boxes are perched on poles in the lake. Soon you'll pass a

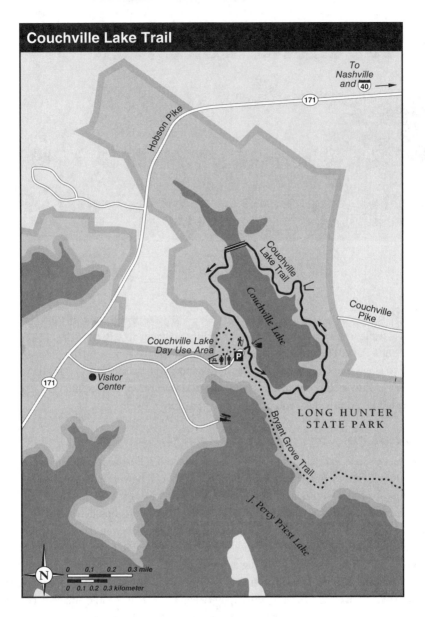

Couchville Lake Trail

sinkhole/pond on your right that was formed in the same manner as Couchville Lake. A smaller pond is just beyond the first.

Circle around the lake and enter a cedar grove. The cedar, which often grows in poor soils, is important for wildlife. Birds use its thin, stringy bark to build nests, songbirds eat its berrylike fruit, and deer feed on its green foliage.

More piers jut into the lake before the trail passes over a dry drainage at mile 1. Ahead are resting benches covered by a shelter that would come in handy during a summer thunderstorm. Look for a willow-rimmed pond to your right, noting that the land

DISTANCE AND CONFIGURATION: 2-mile loop	**MAPS:** USGS *La Vergne*; at **tinyurl.com/longhuntermap**
DIFFICULTY: Easy	**FACILITIES:** Restrooms, water at trailhead
SCENERY: Lakeside forest	**CONTACT:** 615-885-2422; **tnstateparks**
EXPOSURE: Mostly shady	**.com/parks/about/long-hunter**
TRAFFIC: Busy on weekends and weekday afternoons	**LOCATION:** Hermitage
TRAIL SURFACE: Smooth asphalt	**COMMENTS:** This is a barrier-free trail. Couchville Lake is open to fishing. Long Hunter State Park has a fishing pier and rents canoes and small johnboats. No gas motors are allowed, which makes for a more peaceful experience.
HIKING TIME: 1 hour	
ACCESS: No fees or permits required	
PETS: Not allowed on this trail	

bridge between Couchville Lake and the pond is very narrow. These are black willows, the most common of a dozen willows that grow in North America. These trees grow in wet soil along rivers and lakes, acting as a natural erosion barrier. In pioneer days, willow charcoal was a source of gunpowder; nowadays, it is used in furniture, baskets, barrels, and pulpwood. In Middle Tennessee, willow rarely grows to commercial-timber size as it does in the lower Mississippi River Valley.

At mile 1.4, span Couchville Lake on a 300-foot wooden bridge that offers the best lake vistas on the entire trail. Imagine the scene before you as a wooded depression, as it was before J. Percy Priest Lake dam was built. Persimmon trees grow beyond the bridge; look for furrowed bark broken in squares. In the fall, you will see sweet orange persimmon fruit among the leaves and overhead, still on the tree even after its leaves have fallen. This fruit recalls the flavor of dates. Hard, unripe persimmons are unpalatable, though, so make sure to get a softer, riper fruit. In fact, many old-timers believe persimmons shouldn't be eaten until after the first frost. American Indians made persimmon bread and stored the dried fruit like prunes. Opossums, raccoons, skunks, deer, and birds enjoy the fruit, which contains a few seeds. I love persimmons too.

The trail curves around a low drainage to the right, where hackberries grow in a nearly pure stand. These trees, which have gray bark dotted with obvious corky warts, favor moist soil such as this drainage. The trail treads farther from the lake, and dirt paths reach out to more small docks that extend into the water. Just ahead you will find the fishing pier, a picnic area, the boat-rental headquarters, and the end of the loop.

GPS TRAILHEAD COORDINATES
N36° 5.573' W86° 32.618'

From Exit 226 on I-40, east of downtown Nashville, take TN 171 South/South Mount Juliet Road 4.2 miles south. Veer right at the split, as TN 171 becomes Hobson Pike. Continue 2.4 miles, turning left into the Couchville Lake Day Use Area. Continue 0.4 mile and turn left into Area Two. Soon reach the parking area and trailhead. The trail starts near the fishing pier on the edge of Couchville Lake.

4 Ganier Ridge Loop

In Brief

This loop explores the high and the low of Radnor Lake State Park. Depart from the less-used east side of the park, and then climb steeply up the Ganier Ridge Trail into the highest hills in Nashville. Just as you get accustomed to the oak forest up there, the loop drops down to a rich hollow and reaches the north shore of Radnor Lake, a haven for waterfowl. Finish your hike in the flat alongside Radnor Lake.

Description

This hike climbs to about as high as you can get in the Nashville Basin. The areas around it were once simple farms, and the rugged hills have been logged over. But the story of Radnor Lake begins when the Louisville and Nashville Railroad, or L&N, purchased this parcel of land. Back in 1919, the railroad impounded Otter Creek to create Radnor Lake and used its water for steam engines at the adjacent Radnor Yards. The land around the lake was used as a hunting preserve for the elite at L&N. These officials soon recognized the heavy use of the lake by native and migratory birds and declared the area a wildlife sanctuary at the urging of the Tennessee Ornithological Society. Ganier Ridge is named after Albert Ganier, an active member of the society that swayed the L&N to preserve the area. To this day, hikers of this loop can see the small plaque commemorating him. In 1973 the state of Tennessee purchased the 747-acre preserve (now more than 1,300 acres) with the help of citizen donations. The preserve remains an oasis of nature in the middle of Nashville. Birders will enjoy the park's Barbara J. Mapp Aviary Education Center, which houses several birds of prey ranging from great horned owls to bald eagles.

The Access Trail leads into a viny hardwood forest. Climb west with Ganier Ridge to your right. Then descend to reach a trail junction at 0.2 mile. Turn right, passing over a dry branch on a footbridge, and then ascend by switchbacks up Ganier Ridge. Notice the wire fence; this was part of an old farm, one of the early incarnations of the Radnor Lake area. Ganier Ridge is part of the Overton Hills, named for John Overton, one of Nashville's early movers and shakers. He likely once owned the land you are walking on. His home, Travellers Rest, is just east of here off Franklin Pike.

Top out on the ridge in a hickory- and oak-dominated forest. Stay at or near the ridgeline. The walking is glorious among the sometimes windswept hardwoods atop this hill. Swing around to the left side of the actual high point before reaching mile 1 and a contemplation bench that faces the plaque commemorating Albert Ganier. The stone-based memorial is only about 2 feet high and is easily missed. In fact, if it weren't for Ganier we may have missed out entirely on this park. The slight rumbling of autos in the distance belies the wild aura that pulses here.

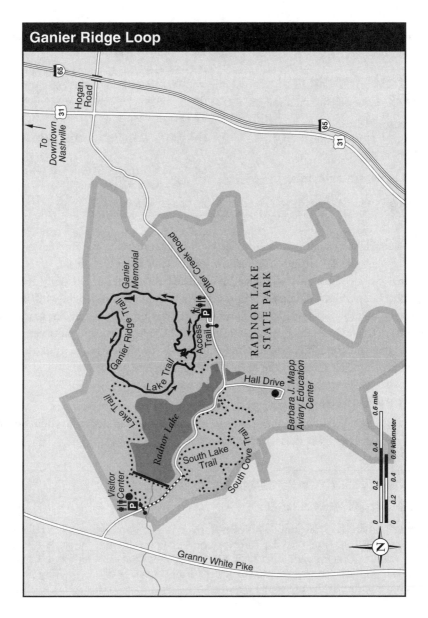

Ganier Ridge Loop

Descend from the plaque, and then turn sharply left down the now rocky ridge. The forest here is more open and stunted, due to the south-facing rocky soil being parched by the sun. This contrasts with the rich cove—into which the Ganier Ridge Trail descends by steps—where hardwoods such as tulip, maple, and sycamore grow tall in the thick, moist soil. Soon, cross an intermittent streambed by bridge to reach an old woods road. The Ganier Ridge Trail turns left here, tracing a carpet of wood chips over what once may have been a logging road. Intersect the Lake Trail at mile 1.7 and stay left, keeping Radnor

DISTANCE AND CONFIGURATION: 2.4-mile loop	**ACCESS:** No fees or permits required; daily, 6 a.m.–sunset
DIFFICULTY: Moderate	**MAPS:** USGS *Oak Hill;* at **tnstateparks .com/assets/pdf/additional-content /park-maps/radnor-lake_area-map.pdf**
SCENERY: Wooded hills and valleys	
EXPOSURE: Shady	**PETS:** On leash only
	FACILITIES: Water spigot, restrooms at trailhead
TRAFFIC: Fairly busy	
TRAIL SURFACE: Dirt, rocks	**CONTACT:** 615-373-3467; **tnstateparks .com/parks/about/radnor-lake**
HIKING TIME: 1.8 hours	**LOCATION:** Nashville

Lake to your right; the impoundment is visible through the trees. The land flattens but is still bisected by small drainages coming down from Ganier Ridge.

You'll cross a substantial drainage by footbridge. Then the trail briefly splits and merges back together. The high road passes by a contemplation bench, while the low road stays along the drainage. Reach another trail junction. Stay left again, as the right trail leads to Otter Creek Road. Ascend a rib ridge of Ganier Ridge and meet yet another junction, one you are familiar with—the beginning of the Ganier Ridge Trail. Keep forward and backtrack 0.2 mile on the Access Trail to complete the loop.

Nearby Activities

The busier west side of the park has a nature center. It has an excellent film about how the park was saved, as well as other nature displays.

GPS TRAILHEAD COORDINATES
N36° 3.482' W86° 47.551'

From Exit 78 on I-65, south of downtown Nashville, take Harding Place 0.4 mile west to intersect US 31/Franklin Pike. Turn left on Franklin Pike and follow it 1.3 miles south to Otter Creek Road. Turn right on Otter Creek Road and follow it 1.2 miles to the parking area on your right. The Access Trail starts beside the parking permit–restroom building at the top of the parking area.

5 Harpeth Woods Trail

In Brief

Part of the Warner Parks trail system, this hike combines human and natural history as it loops through the Harpeth Hills, a collection of ridges southwest of downtown Nashville. First, the Harpeth Woods Trail follows a portion of the old Natchez Trace before visiting a long-abandoned rock quarry in the Little Harpeth River Valley. It then climbs a knob, passing some old-growth trees before descending back along a small stream to once again pick up the old trace. Gravel has been added to the trail base to mitigate heavy use.

Description

This loop makes a great hike for those who don't want to spend an entire day driving to and from the trailhead. Moreover, it offers an escape into the forest and a day's worth of exercise.

First, stop at the covered trailside kiosk near the parking area. Turn right and follow the blue blazes southwest down the straight dirt-and-rock path, which is a remnant of the original Natchez Trace before it was rerouted farther south. More than two centuries old, this trail was considered the "interstate" of travel between Natchez, Mississippi, and Nashville in the early 1800s.

Continuing, you'll span Vaughns Creek on a footbridge. You may walk around the bridge, as Vaughns Creek is most often low or dry at this point. Then keep forward in deep woods, only to leave the old trace and climb a rocky hillside to meet a side trail. Take this short trail to the quarry, where the open brightness offers great contrast to the shadier woods. Stone was first extracted here by settlers of the Little Harpeth River Valley and later by Depression-era workers for the gates and walls you see around the park.

Return to the main trail to bisect a closed paved road, and you'll arrive at a forest heavy with cedar trees. Many of these are large for cedars, but they don't get much acclaim because the large cedars aren't nearly as large as the huge oaks you will eventually pass. The tree canopy breaks open as Harpeth Woods Trail meets Owl Hollow Trail at mile 1.3. This interpretive trail (get an informative booklet about it at the park nature center) circles the valley to your left.

Harpeth Woods Trail continues forward to reach a picnic shelter, near the Little Harpeth River, before ascending a knob via switchbacks that pass the other end of the Owl Hollow Trail along the way. The trail nearly runs into the aforementioned huge oak tree, complete with ferns growing in a crook on the lower limbs. These are known as resurrection ferns, as they curl up when the weather is dry then unfurl and become green after rains; they are more common farther south, especially in Florida.

Leave the ferns behind, cross another paved road (most of Edwin Warner Park's paved roads, once used as scenic drives, are closed to autos and traveled by hikers and

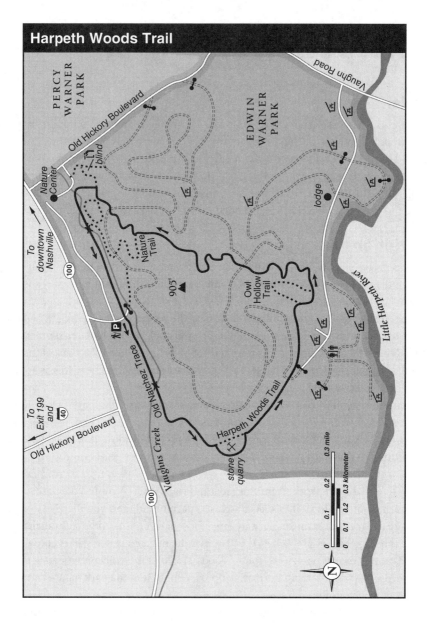

bikers), and keep switchbacking upward to reach the crest of the knob. Work around the knob, which reaches over 900 feet in elevation and stands nearly 300 feet above Vaughns Creek. And stay with the blue blazes, as Harpeth Woods Trail switchbacks downhill to meet the Nature Trail then bisects another closed paved road. You'll approach a huge beech tree beside an intermittent streambed before meeting the old Natchez Trace once again at a trail junction; the path that runs forward will lead you to the nature center. Turn left on the trace and follow the trail to a bridge over Vaughns Creek. At this point

DISTANCE AND CONFIGURATION: 2.5-mile loop	**PETS:** On leash only
DIFFICULTY: Easy	**MAPS:** USGS *Bellevue;* at **tinyurl.com/harpethwoods**
SCENERY: Hardwood and cedar forest, small creek	**FACILITIES:** Restrooms, water at nature center
EXPOSURE: Mostly shady	
TRAFFIC: Busy on weekends	**CONTACT:** 615-352-6299; **tinyurl.com/warnerparknc**
TRAIL SURFACE: Gravel	
HIKING TIME: 1.3 hours	**LOCATION:** Nashville
ACCESS: No fees or permits required; daily, sunrise–11 p.m.	**COMMENTS:** Add Owl Hollow Trail for a 2.8-mile loop.

Vaughns Creek runs perennially, unlike farther downstream where it simply dries up at the surface in late summer and fall. Keep forward on the old trace, with the knob to your left and a field to your right, to shortly complete the loop.

Nearby Activities

The Warner Parks Nature Center is a point of pride for the Nashville park system. It offers wide-ranging environmental education programs for visitors of all ages. Its large learning center has an exhibit hall, outdoor classroom, and more. Also in the area are a library with a large collection of natural-history books, a teaching pond, and a wildflower garden.

GPS TRAILHEAD COORDINATES

N36° 3.542' W86° 54.605'

From Exit 199 on I-40, west of downtown Nashville, take Old Hickory Boulevard 3.8 miles south to intersect TN 100. Turn left on TN 100 and follow it 0.3 mile to the Edwin Warner Park trailhead, on your right. Turn right, and then park in the trailhead parking to the right. The blue-blazed path starts near the trail kiosk.

6 Jones Mill Trail

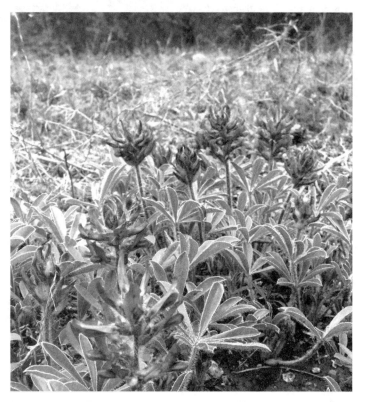

Larkspur colors a trailside clearing.

In Brief

This popular trail in the Bryant Grove area of Long Hunter State Park was designed by mountain bikers but welcomes hikers. It travels through open cedar glades, gravel glades, and cedar forests along the shores of J. Percy Priest Lake. Avoid it on weekend afternoons.

Description

After leaving the large parking area, you'll immediately come to the first loop of the hike. Stay left here on a singletrack path, traveling the typical cedar glade woodland that comprises much of Long Hunter State Park. However, worldwide, the cedar glade is a rare environment, and we as Tennesseans should appreciate every square foot of it. The woodland floor and trail bed are quite stony, but the hickories, cedars, and oaks manage to find their place, as do boxwood bushes and moss in ultrashady spots deep in cedar thickets.

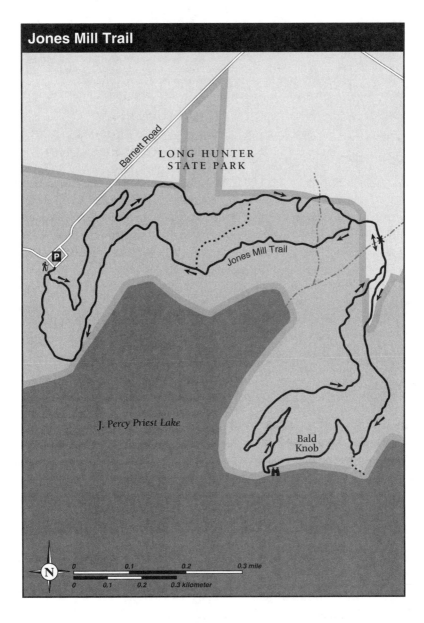

The path runs along a hillside roughly parallel with the lakeshore below. Make a pair of switchbacks starting at 0.3 mile; then resume a northeasterly course amid trees stunted by thin, poor soil and excessive rock, and drift through open glades. At an intersection at 0.7 mile, a shortcut leads right, but the main trail continues in an open glade. Note the old fence line. Woods and glades are interspersed. Be sure to stay on the trail when traveling through these open glades. Despite their appearance, they are a fragile ecosystem harboring rare plants.

DISTANCE AND CONFIGURATION: 3.6-mile figure eight	**HIKING TIME:** 2 hours
	ACCESS: No fees or permits required
DIFFICULTY: Moderate	**MAPS:** USGS *La Vergne;*
SCENERY: Cedar glades, lake, cedar forest	at **tinyurl.com/longhuntermap**
EXPOSURE: Mostly shady	**FACILITIES:** None
TRAFFIC: Heavy with bikes on weekends	**CONTACT:** 615-885-2422; **tnstateparks .com/parks/about/long-hunter**
TRAIL SURFACE: Dirt, roots, rocks, leaves	**LOCATION:** Mount Juliet

Step over a wet-weather drainage at 0.8 mile. At 0.9 mile, you'll reach the other end of the first loop. That will be your return route. Continue toward Bald Knob to cut through a stone fence and span a drainage via a bridge. Reach the second loop at 1.1 miles—continue straight toward Bald Knob. At 1.3 miles, you may see a junction in the future, as Jones Mill Trail is being extended. Begin curving toward J. Percy Priest Lake in a mixed cedar forest with a grassy understory. At 1.5 miles, a faint path leads to the shore, while the main trail curves away from the lake and climbs near the crest of Bald Knob. At 1.6 miles, you'll come alongside a steeply sloped hill and shortly reach a cleared vista of the Hurricane Creek arm of J. Percy Priest Lake.

Switchback off the knob, still on a singletrack path, and pass through a glade at 2.2 miles and open stone slabs. Complete the Bald Knob loop at 2.5 miles, and then backtrack to the trailhead loop, reaching it at 2.7 miles. Veer left into cedars and cover new terrain as you head back toward the parking area, bisecting another stone fence to pass the shortcut's south end at 2.9 miles. Wildflowers are thick here; you'll see shooting stars, phlox, and larkspur, among others. You'll pass near the water at 3.4 miles. At low water, you can access a gravel beach down here by simply aiming for the lake. The maintained trail abruptly turns away and heads toward the trailhead, which you reach at 3.6 miles.

Nearby Activities

Long Hunter State Park has a lake and fishing pier, and rents canoes and small johnboats. No gas motors are allowed, which makes for a peaceful experience.

GPS TRAILHEAD COORDINATES

N36° 4.473' W86° 30.591'

From Exit 226 on I-40, east of downtown Nashville, take TN 171 South/South Mount Juliet Road 4.3 miles south. Stay left at the split with Hobson Pike, traveling 1.1 miles farther to hit a T intersection and Couchville Pike. Turn left at the T onto Couchville Pike and follow it 2 miles to Barnett Road. Turn right on Barnett Road and travel 0.4 mile. Turn left into the trailhead parking area.

7 MetroCenter Levee Greenway

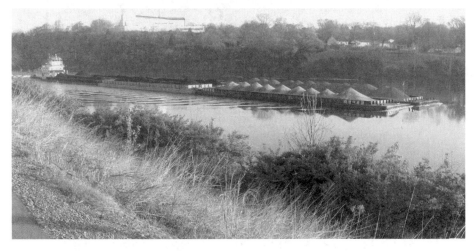

A loaded barge as seen from the MetroCenter Levee Greenway

In Brief

This elevated greenway travels atop a U.S. Army Corps of Engineers–built levee and provides a pleasant venue near downtown Nashville. Don't let its urban setting deter you from checking it out.

Description

I admit to being skeptical before trying this trail. However, after doing it, I give it a ringing endorsement. This 3.5-mile path has been connected to downtown Nashville, expanding the greenway system of the metro area. The story of this greenway begins in the early 1970s when the U.S. Army Corps of Engineers built a levee to protect the flats beside the river here, so businesses could develop. In the 1990s the Corps determined the levee needed to be raised to meet new flood-control standards. The city and the Corps worked together to develop this trail along the improved levee. After a cost of $7.5 million, the trail was completed, opened, and ultimately expanded to link to the heart of downtown. Walkers, runners, and bicyclists all enjoy this path. Many employees of adjacent businesses use the trail at lunchtime.

The well-manicured trailhead serves greenway users heading along the MetroCenter Levee and the greenway heading into downtown Nashville. This trek heads toward the

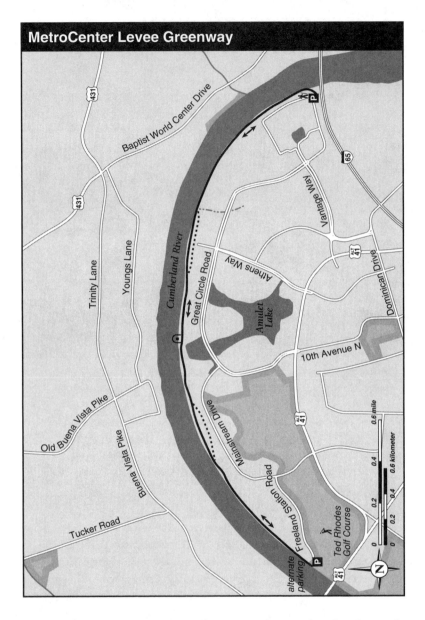

MetroCenter Levee Greenway

river, then joins the levee as it goes away from I-65. The paved trail is about 8 feet wide and roughly parallels the shoreline of the Cumberland River. Interesting shaded rest stops incorporate aquatic art reflecting the water. Art is also integrated into the concrete flood-wall, the decorative trailside fences, and even the pavement.

Travel the path resting atop a berm straddling the margin between businesses to your left and the Cumberland River to your right. Make no mistake—this isn't a wilder-ness hike, but it is a not-to-be-overlooked exercise venue. Think of it as a way of varying your outdoor experiences. Be prepared for open conditions, as shade is short. Brush,

DISTANCE AND CONFIGURATION: 5.8-mile out-and-back	**ACCESS:** No fees or permits required
DIFFICULTY: Moderate due to distance	**PETS:** Yes
SCENERY: Cumberland River, businesses and offices	**MAPS:** USGS *Nashville West;* at **greenwaysfornashville.org/PDFmaps /CumberlandRiver.pdf**
EXPOSURE: Mostly sunny	**FACILITIES:** None
TRAFFIC: Moderate	**CONTACT:** 615-862-8400; **nashville.gov/Parks-and-Recreation**
TRAIL SURFACE: Asphalt	
HIKING TIME: 2.5 hours	**LOCATION:** Nashville

riprap, and some trees—hackberry and sycamore—extend toward the river. Cotton-woods are also prevalent. The far shoreline is populated with occasional houses and businesses atop bluffs and hills.

At 0.9 mile, the levee splits, and you have a trail that runs closer to the river. Take this lower path, which soon rejoins the main levee trail. At 1.5 miles, you'll arrive at a "new-fashioned" covered bridge. The 150-foot cylindrical screen tunnel through which you pass actually serves to hide a water-pumping station. This is also part of the integrated functional art found along the greenway. Landward views here include Amulet Lake.

At 1.8 miles, the trail splits again. Take the route that descends toward the river to enjoy the only shady section of trail. The paths rejoin at 2.2 miles, and you're once again atop the levee. The trail now curves southwest and soon reaches the Freeland Station Road trailhead at 2.9 miles. In case you want to just go one way and use a shuttle from the Great Circle Road trailhead, take Great Circle Road to Mainstream Drive. Turn right on Mainstream Drive, then take another right onto Freeland Station Road and follow it to dead-end at this western trailhead.

Nearby Activities

Use the Great Circle Road trailhead to access downtown Nashville via a greenway connecting to the already-built portions of greater Cumberland River Greenway in the heart of Music City.

GPS TRAILHEAD COORDINATES
N36° 11.537' W86° 47.117'

From Exit 85 (Alt US 41/State Capitol/Rosa L. Parks Boulevard) on I-65 near downtown, take Alt US 41 North toward MetroCenter. Follow Alt US 41/Rosa L. Parks Boulevard north 0.4 mile to Vantage Way. Turn right on Vantage Way and follow it 0.5 mile. Turn right on Great Circle Road and follow it 0.3 mile to dead-end at the trailhead, near the I-65 overpass spanning the Cumberland River.

8 Mill Creek Greenway

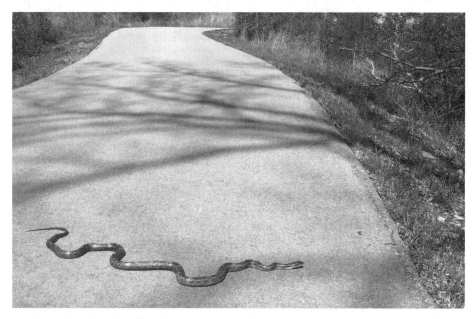

Even snakes like the Mill Creek Greenway.

In Brief

This greenway is an urban classic, tucked away in a heavily developed area of Antioch adjacent to I-24. It uses not only lands along the surprisingly pretty Mill Creek but also public property on the edge of Antioch Middle School and Antioch Community Center.

Description

Mill Creek is doing its best to remain a beautiful stream. In fact, the water coloration is still bluish, and paddlers can be found plying Mill Creek in spring and early summer. You arrived here on Blue Hole Road, named for a deep spot in the creek that has an especially deep-blue cast. A canoe-manufacturing company, Blue Hole Canoe, was named after this stream.

This walk begins on Whittemore Branch, a feeder stream of Mill Creek located behind the trailhead kiosk. From here, turn left and head upstream, with the creek to your right and Antioch Community Center to your left; I-24 is noisily close.

The greenway begins circling around the community center to pass under Blue Hole Road. A field and play area are located adjacent to the community center. The trail then squeezes behind Antioch Middle School, which longtime Antioch residents recall was once Antioch High School. Soon you'll saddle alongside Mill Creek to your right. Look over the

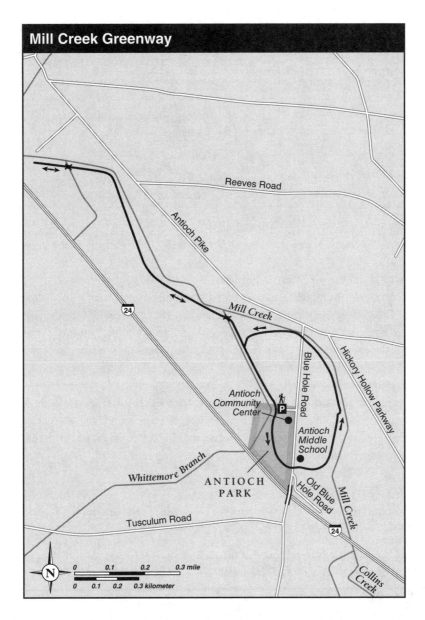

Mill Creek Greenway

Reeves Road

Antioch Pike

24

Mill Creek

Antioch Community Center

Blue Hole Road

Hickory Hollow Parkway

Antioch Middle School

Whittemore Branch

ANTIOCH PARK

Old Blue Hole Road

Mill Creek

24

Tusculum Road

Collins Creek

N

0   0.1   0.2   0.3 mile

0   0.1   0.2   0.3 kilometer

creek's still-bluish cast. At 0.6 mile, the trail passes beneath Blue Hole Road again, this time under a bridge spanning Mill Creek. When the creek floods, this part of the greenway can become muddy, though the trail is scraped clean by the city as soon as the water recedes.

The greenway continues along Mill Creek to complete the loop portion of the walk at 0.8 mile. Turn right, continuing downstream along Mill Creek. In days long past, early Nashvillians set up a gristmill on this stream, using water power to grind corn into meal, giving the stream its name. The greenway spans a feeder stream on a sturdy iron bridge,

DISTANCE AND CONFIGURATION: 2.6-mile loop plus out-and-back	**ACCESS:** No fees or permits required
DIFFICULTY: Easy	**PETS:** Yes
SCENERY: Urban interface, streamside woods	**MAPS:** USGS *Antioch;* at **greenwaysfor nashville.org/PDFmaps/MillCreek.pdf**
EXPOSURE: More sun than shade	**FACILITIES:** Restrooms at Antioch Community Center
TRAFFIC: Moderate–heavy on weekends	**CONTACT:** 615-862-8400; **nashville.gov /Parks-and-Recreation**
TRAIL SURFACE: Paved	
HIKING TIME: 1.75 hours	**LOCATION:** Antioch

then climbs a bit of a hill as it works around a bluff. This segment of the greenway is more shaded.

Even though the greenway is bordered by civilization on both sides, it still offers refuge for wildlife, even snakes, as shown in the accompanying photo. Greenways such as this one, situated along a stream, protect wetlands and help with flood control, thanks to preserved and nonchannelized streams that absorb excess runoff. Continue downstream and enjoy the scenery as you pass a second bridge at 1.5 miles; the stream traveling underneath also feeds Mill Creek. Just ahead, at 1.6 miles, the Mill Creek Greenway currently ends. It is 1 mile back to the trailhead.

Keep apprised, as this greenway is being extended. Greenways such as this provide community benefits, and you will see many people exercising along the path. And as Nashville's greenway system becomes more extended and connected, its paths will be used as transportation corridors.

Nearby Activities

Two additional but noncontiguous segments of the Mill Creek Greenway have been completed near Ezell Park and Mill Creek Park.

GPS TRAILHEAD COORDINATES

N36° 3.440' W86° 40.403'

From Exit 59 (Bell Road) on I-24, southeast of downtown Nashville, take Bell Road west 0.8 mile to Blue Hole Road. Turn right on Blue Hole Road and follow it 0.7 mile to reach the Antioch Community Center. The greenway starts at the back of the parking area.

9 Mossy Ridge Trail

In Brief

Mossy Ridge Trail is the longest of the three loop footpaths in the Warner Parks. It is the quietest and least used loop as well. An ideal training hike, the path leaves the Deep Well trailhead and winds through rich hollows and dry ridges of the Harpeth Hills, making frequent but never sustained elevation changes. Scattered in the woods are big trees and a spring-fed waterfall.

Description

At 4.5 miles, Mossy Ridge Trail qualifies as a full-fledged hike that will not disappoint. If it weren't for some park road crossings and a little noise from TN 100, hikers would think they were in a remote swath of Middle Tennessee back in the days when Nashvillians traveled by horse. You will be traveling by foot in cove hardwood forests and along hickory–oak–cedar ridges in Percy Warner Park, where the hiking rivals any city park in the country.

Leave the covered trailside kiosk and trace the red blazes to a trail junction, crossing the wide, Old Beech bridle path for the first of many times. Warner Woods Trail goes left, and Mossy Ridge Trail goes right, swinging alongside a hillside outcropped with mossy rocks. Look to your right at a spring below. Soon you'll reach a second junction at 0.1 mile; the loop portion of Mossy Ridge Trail begins here.

Turn right, crossing the bridle path, and descend to a hollow rich with tulip trees before reaching a side trail at 0.5 mile. This trail leads right 70 yards on a surprisingly narrow ridgeline to a bench at Quiet Point. Mossy Ridge Trail keeps forward and climbs to meet a scenic park road on Gum Ridge. The path drops along the north side of the ridge into Dripping Spring Hollow. Here a spring seep drops over an exposed rock line to make a wet-weather waterfall. The trail is slippery as it bridges the exposed rock line, so consider taking the Dripping Spring Bypass, which skirts below the rock line and the wet-weather waterfall to meet the main trail. The path then winds above Ginger Hollow and Dome Hollow and

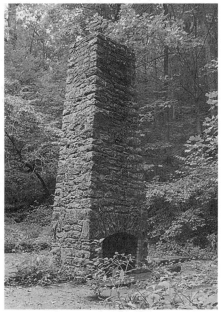

Chimney from the Betsy Ross cabin

39

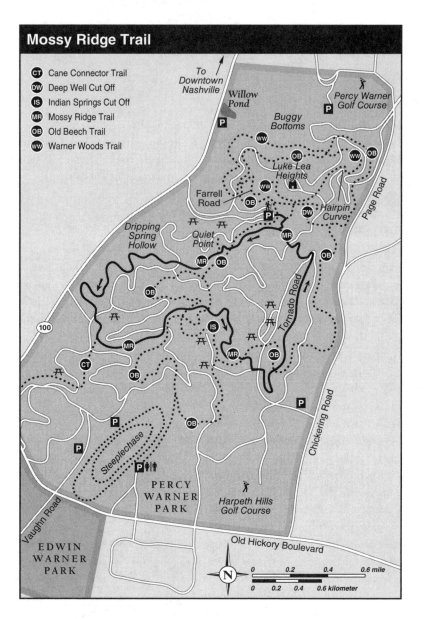

Mossy Ridge Trail

- **CT** Cane Connector Trail
- **DW** Deep Well Cut Off
- **IS** Indian Springs Cut Off
- **MR** Mossy Ridge Trail
- **OB** Old Beech Trail
- **WW** Warner Woods Trail

To Downtown Nashville

Willow Pond

Buggy Bottoms

Percy Warner Golf Course

Luke Lea Heights

Farrell Road

Hairpin Curve

Dripping Spring Hollow

Quiet Point

Page Road

100

Tornado Road

Chickering Road

Steeplechase

PERCY WARNER PARK

Harpeth Hills Golf Course

Vaughn Road

EDWIN WARNER PARK

Old Hickory Boulevard

N

0   0.2   0.4   0.6 mile
0   0.2   0.4   0.6 kilometer

descends by long switchbacks to near TN 100. A field is visible beyond the line of woods. Cross another park road before reaching a junction with Cane Connector Trail at mile 1.9. This trail leads right and connects to the trails at adjacent Edwin Warner Park.

The ups and downs continue as Mossy Ridge Trail ascends the side of what is now known as Mossy Ridge, where moss carpets the ground below scattered oaks, cedar, and rocks. Stay on the ridgeline to cross a park road. Then follow the red blazes of the footpath, but don't pick up the horse trail, which also crosses the road. Soon cross the bridle path twice in succession, and ascend to a hilltop known as Rattlesnake Circle. Make easy

DISTANCE AND CONFIGURATION: 4.5-mile loop	**ACCESS:** No fees or permits required; daily, sunrise–11 p.m.
DIFFICULTY: Moderate	**PETS:** On leash only
SCENERY: Woodlands	**MAPS:** USGS *Bellevue;* at **tinyurl.com/mossyridgetrl**
EXPOSURE: Nearly all shady	
TRAFFIC: Moderate on weekends, some noise from TN 100	**FACILITIES:** Portable restroom at Deep Well trailhead
TRAIL SURFACE: Dirt, some rocks	**CONTACT:** 615-352-6299; **tinyurl.com/warnerparknc**
HIKING TIME: 2.3 hours	**LOCATION:** Nashville

tracks among both spindly and large trees. Drop to near the Indian Springs Picnic Area. Reach a paved road and turn left on the road, bridging a streambed. Cross a road and a mowed field before reentering forestland. Make a long switchback, working up to the ridgeline known as Tornado Road, where the trailside is adorned with the first tree-identification signs. The walking is easy here. The next ridgeline over to the east is visible. And Tornado Road ends all too soon as it drops to a paved park road. Turn left, following the paved park road, veer right, and drop into Basswood Hollow.

Middle Tennessee is near the southern end of the basswood's growth range. This tree's roundish leaves are almost as wide as they are long, and its bark becomes furrowed as it ages. Sharply climb out of Basswood Hollow to cross a paved road and drop into another hollow where a chimney stands. This is a relic of the Betsy Ross Cabin, which was built by Boy Scouts in the 1930s. Continue down the hollow past the cabin site to soon reach the beginning of Mossy Ridge Trail. From here, backtrack a short distance to the Deep Well trailhead.

Nearby Activities

Warner Parks Nature Center is a point of pride for the Nashville park system. It offers wide-ranging environmental-education programs for visitors of all ages. Its large learning center has an exhibit hall, outdoor classroom, and more. Also in the area are a library with a large collection of natural-history books, a teaching pond, and a wildflower garden.

GPS TRAILHEAD COORDINATES

N36° 4.703' W86° 52.790'

From the point where TN 100 begins at US 70S near the Belle Meade Post Office, head west on TN 100 for 1.7 miles to the large stone gates on the left that mark the Deep Well entrance of Percy Warner Park. Turn left from TN 100 and pass through the gates, staying right when the road splits. Reach the Deep Well trailhead parking at 0.6 mile. Mossy Ridge Trail starts behind the trailside kiosk.

10 Old Hickory Lake Nature Trail

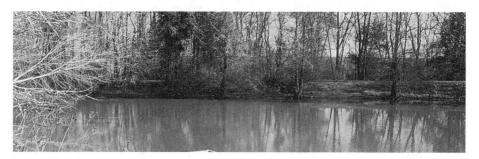

The all-access pond on Old Hickory Lake Nature Trail

In Brief

This easy walk, suitable for young children, uses a combination of three miniloops to explore the woods near Old Hickory Lake Dam. The loops traverse pine woods and go over boardwalks, culminating in a trip to a pond with a viewing platform.

Description

This trail is actually part of the Nashville Greenway system, though only a portion of the path is paved. The U.S. Army Corps of Engineers built it in the mid-1970s. The mounds you see in the area are part of the dredging material left from the erection of nearby Old Hickory Dam, which was finished in 1954. The forest has reclaimed the area, with the help of some loblolly pines planted in the 1960s.

The loblolly pine is not native to Middle Tennessee (it grows in a belt from east Texas to Florida and north to eastern Virginia) and is among the fastest-growing Southern pines. The pine's rapid growth makes it popular for planting and cultivation for pulpwood and lumber. Even by pine standards, the loblolly has especially fragrant needles.

The manner in which nature repairs itself is called plant succession. For example, an area is cleared and then covered with fill. Later, plants that thrive in the sun, such as black-berries, begin to grow. These species provide shade for young plants and trees that can't tolerate open sun. The trees then grow and ultimately return the forest to its former state.

Leave the parking area and soon enter Woodland Loop. Circle through loblolly pines, passing beneath a power line. A viewing blind is to your left. Quietly head over to the fence and peer through the boards, where a deer or squirrel may be stirring. Reach a long board-walk that winds over a wetland. To protect them from drainage and development, wetlands have come under increasing protection over the years. Wetlands are natural filters for water as it seeps into the earth, and also foster wildlife and insects, especially mosquitoes.

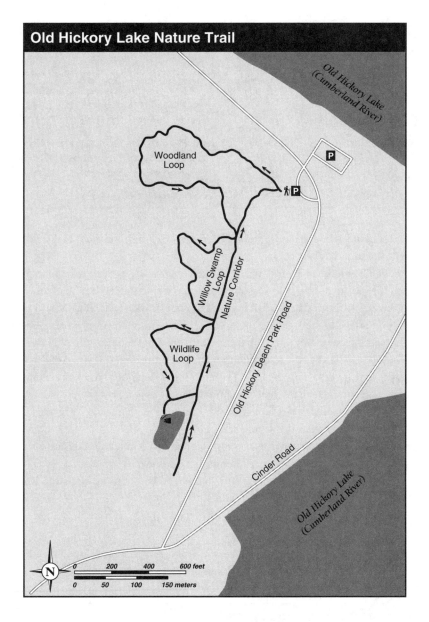

Old Hickory Lake Nature Trail

Leave the Woodland Loop at 0.4 mile, near the main paved path. Return to the woods, now on the Willow Swamp Loop. Soon reach another boardwalk. Willow trees thrive where drainage is poor, claiming their special niche in the web of life. Sycamore trees also grow along the wetter margins. In summer, the swamp emits the pungent odor of decay.

Return to the paved part of the trail, but soon turn away on the Wildlife Loop. This trail curves beneath the tall pines—notice the blackened trunks of trees here. Low-level, low-intensity forest fires often sweep through pine woods. To thrive and ultimately

DISTANCE AND CONFIGURATION: 1.5-mile triple loop	ACCESS: No fees or permits required
DIFFICULTY: Easy	MAPS: USGS *Goodlettsville;* at trailhead
SCENERY: Pine and hardwood forest, willow swamp, pond	PETS: On leash only
EXPOSURE: Nearly all shady	FACILITIES: Restrooms at nearby swim beach
TRAFFIC: Some	CONTACT: 615-736-7161; **www.lrn .usace.army.mil/Locations/Lakes/Old HickoryLake/Recreation/Trails.aspx**
TRAIL SURFACE: Asphalt, pine needles, boardwalks	
HIKING TIME: 1 hour	LOCATION: Old Hickory

survive, a pine forest needs periodic fire. Some species of pine, such as Florida's sand pine, need fire to open their cones.

Soon you'll emerge at a pond, where a little viewing platform allows you to peer into the water. Life at the pond varies season to season. During winter, a time of hibernation, frogs and turtles lie buried in the soil beneath the pond, and toads, snakes, and salamanders will be under old stumps and logs. Spring, though, is much more alive. Birds are singing. Ducks may be swimming. Turtles are out, enjoying the sun atop old logs. In summer, the pond may be abuzz with dragonflies chasing mosquitoes. If you come here in the evening, crickets by the thousands will be humming in harmony, and lightning bugs will be flickering off and on. Fall is when the pond will be at its lowest. Decaying leaves will be floating on the surface, later to enhance the nutrients of the pond. And marsh plants around the pond move in as the water shallows.

Follow the paved path from the viewing platform to the main paved Nature Corridor. If you go to the right, the trail soon dead-ends, but you can circle the pond on an informal path. To the left, the paved trail leads through the woods past more wetlands. Enjoy this last relaxing stroll before reaching the trailhead.

Nearby Activities

Old Hickory Beach is open in the warm season, is a year-round boat launch, and has picnic areas and a playground. For more information, call 615-822-4846.

GPS TRAILHEAD COORDINATES
N36° 17.708' W86° 39.413'

From Exit 92 on I-65, north of downtown Nashville, take TN 45 4 miles east to Robinson Road, which is just after the bridge crossing the Cumberland River. Turn left on Bridgeway Avenue and follow it 0.5 mile to Swinging Bridge Road. Turn left on Swinging Bridge Road and follow it 1.2 miles to Cinder Road. Turn right on Cinder Road and follow it 0.8 mile to reach Old Hickory Lake. Turn left at the sign for Old Hickory Lake Nature Trail, which will be on your left at 0.4 mile.

11 Peeler Park Hike

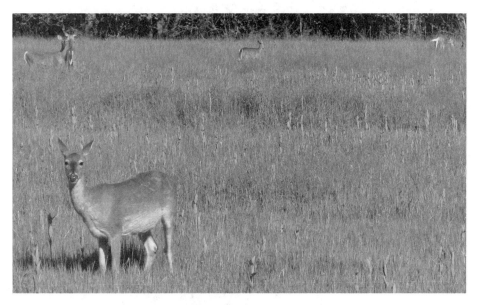

The meadows of Peeler Park attract trailside deer.

In Brief

One of Nashville's newer parks has gotten better with the addition of natural-surface hiking trails complementing the original greenway. Now hikers can use a mix of paved, gravel, and natural-surface paths to make an exploratory loop through a serene natural area of fields, hills, wetlands, and woods along the Cumberland River.

Description

This hike, located near Madison, is more proof that the city of Nashville is once again turning to the Cumberland River, the reason for its location in the first place. Peeler Park is set on the inside of Neelys Bend at the end of a dead-end road. The city first acquired the property back in 1963, from a farmer by the name of E. N. Peeler. The city held onto the land and subsequently bought the adjacent property of Sun Valley Swim Club in 1969. For years, the land was leased out as a farm. More than a generation passed before the city began to develop the park and open it for use. The resultant trail system is gaining in popularity, but the majority of users come from nearby Madison. I suggest a spring or fall afternoon to explore this swath of green space that features not only the river but also wetlands recalling the Deep South more than Middle Tennessee. Note: A separate set of trails is open to equestrians, but hikers and cyclists

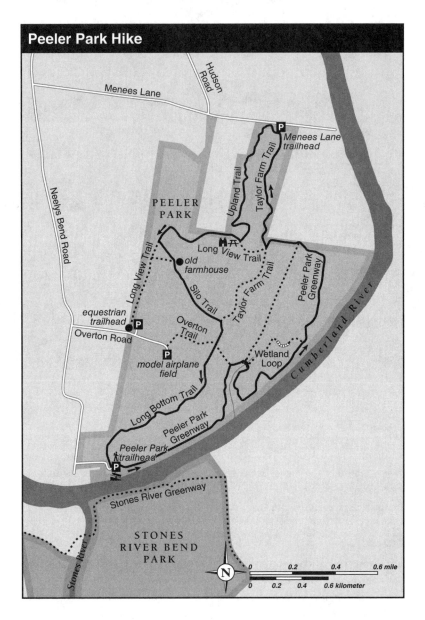

Peeler Park Hike

are expressly prohibited from using the bridle paths, so don't tempt fate—stick with the hiker-only trails.

Trail users are greeted with a first-rate trailhead, complete with a shaded gazebo, metal benches, and a color map of Peeler Park. Your hike will be on asphalt greenway at first. Natural-surface trails return you to the trailhead. Join the Peeler Park Greenway as it heads upstream on the northwest bank of the Cumberland River. A line of thick trees, cane, and brush divides you from the water about 40 feet below. To your left, a slender

DISTANCE AND CONFIGURATION: 5.5-mile loop	**ACCESS:** No fees or permits required
DIFFICULTY: Moderate	**PETS:** On leash only
SCENERY: Fields and woods, wetlands, Cumberland River	**MAPS:** USGS *Nashville East;* at **greenwaysfornashville.org/maps-trails /sm_files/peeler.pdf**
EXPOSURE: Half sunny, half shady	**FACILITIES:** Boat ramp at trailhead
TRAFFIC: Moderate	
TRAIL SURFACE: Asphalt, gravel, grass, natural surface	**CONTACT:** 615-862-8400; **nashville.gov/Parks-and-Recreation**
HIKING TIME: 3 hours	**LOCATION:** Madison

field runs parallel with the path. Equestrians access their paths from a separate trailhead. Expect to see deer and turkey somewhere along this hike.

Contemplation benches are scattered along the path. Travel under an open sky, walking the nexus between field and forest. Occasional spur paths lead to clearings overlooking the Cumberland. After 0.25 mile, you'll reach a park-built path leading to the river. Stones River Greenway runs on the other side of the Cumberland. Peeler Park Greenway turns away from the river at 0.6 mile, now drifting into woodland bordering a tributary. The feeder stream cuts a deep ravine at this point. At 0.8 mile, the Overton Trail leads left to Overton Road and the park's model airplane field. Stay right. The trail bridges the creek you've been paralleling, and the ravine is no longer. Stay right to reach a second intersection, now on the paved Wetland Loop.

Begin cruising past a wetland swamp, with buttressed trees rising from the water. The Cumberland River is through the trees to your right. At 1.5 miles, the Wetland Loop heads left over the wetland boardwalk. Stay right, still with the Peeler Park Greenway. Keep north, slowly separating from the river. This part of the park was the most recently developed. Pass through massive meadows mixed with trees. Climb a bit of a hill before reaching a trail junction at 2.2 miles. Here, the Long View Trail goes straight, but you turn right on pea gravel Taylor Farm Trail, resuming the northbound track through alternating fields and lines of trees.

At 2.8 miles, come within sight of the Menees Lane trailhead, but turn left on the hiker-only, grassy Upland Trail. And it does go up. Climb into a mosaic of field and forest, turning south. Stay off any equestrian paths. Sometimes the hiker trails are hard to find, especially where mowed trail meets woods and the path devolves to a slender dirt track. Be patient and watchful at these edges. Continue opening into and out of fields, still southbound. You'll open on and off fields and woods, this time southbound. At 3.6 miles, in an open grassy hill with a view to the east, meet the Long View Trail. Head right, west, still climbing. Pass a picnic table and a view toward the Cumberland River. Keep climbing to reach a high point at 4 miles, shortly after crossing an equestrian-only path. Turn southwest, walking through open terrain to turn left on the Silo Trail at 4.1 miles.

View a bit of history at 4.2 miles, passing an old farmhouse and outbuildings. These may be torn down in the future. Descend a long, grassy hill, and then leave right on the gravel Taylor Farm Trail to reach a four-way intersection at 4.6 miles. Stay straight, joining the Long Bottom Trail. This natural-surface path weaves through wooded swamps and dry woods running alongside them. Hopefully, boardwalks will be installed in the future, as segments traverse true wetlands. Adventurous hikers will work their way through this attractive and botanically diverse area, getting their hiking shoes soaked until the boardwalks are built and reaching the Peeler Park trailhead at 5.5 miles.

Nearby Activities

Use Peeler Park as a takeout for a fantastic urban paddle trip down the Stones River from J. Percy Priest Dam. It is 7 miles of cold water floating past big bluffs in a surprisingly relaxed setting.

GPS TRAILHEAD COORDINATES

N36° 11.693' W86° 39.617'

From Exit 14A (US 31E/Gallatin Road/Madison) on Briley Parkway, on the north side of Nashville, take US 31E 1.5 miles north to Neelys Bend Road. Turn right on Neelys Bend Road and follow it 6 miles. Turn left into Peeler Park and dead-end at the trailhead and a boat ramp on the Cumberland River.

12 Richland Creek Greenway: McCabe Loop

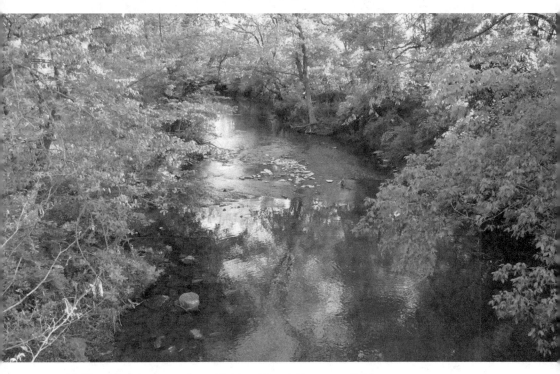

Richland Creek as seen from Richland Creek Greenway Bridge

In Brief

This urban trek, popular with joggers and exercising professionals in the morning and evening, travels along Richland Creek while making a circuit around McCabe Golf Course. With multiple trailheads and spurs connecting to neighborhoods and shopping centers, all integrated into urban Nashville, this trail network both embodies the evolution of the modern greenway and contains a piece of Nashville's past.

Description

Nashville has done an excellent job of integrating its greenways into the existing infrastructure, working trails along creeks, along roads, and in previously established parks, even those with golf courses. The Richland Creek Greenway has been a smashing success

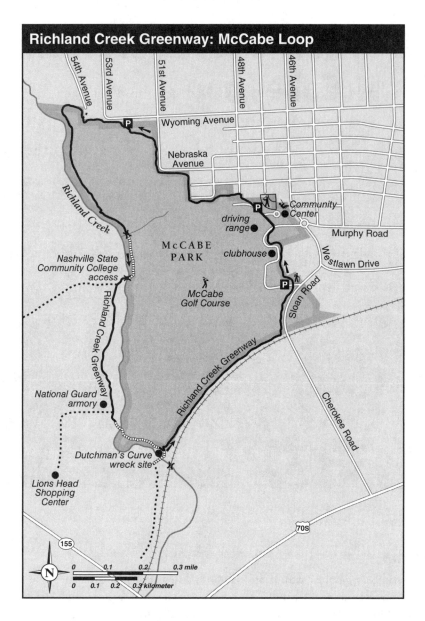

Richland Creek Greenway: McCabe Loop

and is very popular, almost to the point where a golfer hitting an errant shot at McCabe Golf Course blames his misguided swings at the constant circling of hikers, dog walkers, joggers, and bicyclists. No matter; residents of Sylvan Park and other immediate locals use the trail, as do area professionals on break, in addition to curious hikers like us trying to hike all the trails in metro Nashville. Multiple trailheads connect not only Sylvan Park but also the Nashville State Community College (locally known as Nashville Tech) campus, Lions Head, and even the Publix store on Harding Pike.

DISTANCE AND CONFIGURATION: 2.8-mile loop	**ACCESS:** No fees or permits required
DIFFICULTY: Easy–moderate	**PETS:** On leash only
SCENERY: Golf course, stream	**MAPS:** USGS *Nashville West;* at **greenwaysfornashville.org/maps-trails /sm_files/richland.pdf**
EXPOSURE: Half shady	
TRAFFIC: Busy on nice weather weekends, mornings, and evenings	**FACILITIES:** Golf course clubhouse near trailhead
TRAIL SURFACE: Asphalt, concrete	**CONTACT:** 615-862-8400; **nashville.gov/Parks-and-Recreation**
HIKING TIME: 1.5 hours	**LOCATION:** Nashville

While the greenway does loop around a golf course, it has some scenic natural moments, especially where it crosses Richland Creek on footbridges and boardwalks over wetlands. Then, for a moment, you can view the mosaic of land and water that originally drew residents to live here in Music City.

And then there is the accident. Part of the trail passes by the site of the deadliest train crash in American history at a place called Dutchman's Curve. Richland Creek Greenway has a short spur leading to the trestles where it occurred, right next to the current CSX track. This was the old Bosley Road underpass, over which two trains collided that fateful July day in 1918. The overnight express from Memphis heading east to Nashville, part of the NC & St. Louis Railway, was running late, over half an hour behind schedule, and was making up time, hurtling toward Tennessee's capital city. Meanwhile, the local train running from Nashville to Memphis was westbound on the same track. It was running 10 minute late, having left at 7 a.m. Normally, the local train would pull aside on a parallel track at Centennial Park and let the overnight express from Memphis pass, but this time it did not. We do not know why.

The two trains struck head on with a combined speed over 100 miles per hour. All 14 railroad engineers were killed. One of them, Bill Lloyd, was to retire the next day. Over 100 passengers perished, and 100 more were injured. Fires broke out along the line of cars. The death and destruction amazed the thousands who crowded around the chaotic site, hampering rescue efforts. It was truly a dark day for Nashville and the railroad industry.

The Dutchman's Curve wreck site occurs in the second half of the hike. Start the trek at the entrance to McCabe Golf Course, where a circular trailhead contains a map and kiosk. You will first pass behind the golf course clubhouse, then head behind the McCabe Driving Range. Keep your eyes peeled for signs marking the greenway, when it nears sidewalks and parking areas. At 0.3 mile, the greenway comes near the 48th Avenue access and continues tracing the margin between the golf course and the adjacent Sylvan Park neighborhood. At 0.8 mile, the greenway reaches the Wyoming Avenue trailhead. It offers alternate parking.

Beyond the Wyoming access, the Richland Creek Greenway heads west, passing the 54th Avenue entrance at 1 mile, then turns south along Richland Creek. The canopied, rocky stream is heading north to meet the Cumberland River near Bells Bend. Short spur trails lead to the water's edge, and streamside vegetation can be ultradense in summer. Houses rise on the far side of the creek. At 1.5 miles, bridge a channeled tributary draining the golf course and flowing into Richland Creek. The trail then rises to join an elevated boardwalk. Here, an iron footbridge crosses the creek, leading hikers to a trail junction on its west bank. At this point, a spur leads west to the Nashville Tech campus, while the Richland Creek Greenway turns south, traveling well above the waterway below. Pass a National Guard armory, and then meet the spur leaving to the Lions Head trailhead at 2 miles. Now comes a scenic stretch as the trail dips to bridge Richland Creek again. Look downstream for bluffs above the stream. Travel a boardwalk through bottomland. Ahead, a rocky gravel bar of the creek is easily accessible from the trail. At 2.2 miles, a spur goes right to bridge Richland Creek and leads to the trailhead at Publix on US 70S/ Harding Road. Walk out to the bridge, grabbing one last look at Richland Creek; then resume the trek, quickly reaching the train wreck site at Dutchman's Curve. Walk beneath the trestles and soak in the interpretive information. The final stretch leaves Richland Creek and surmounts a hill. At 2.7 miles, turn north, continuing to trace the golf course. Stroll under a mix of trail and tree, returning to the trailhead at 2.8 miles.

Nearby Activities

Richland Creek Greenway encircles McCabe Golf Course, and its connector paths link to all manner of shopping and dining.

GPS TRAILHEAD COORDINATES

N36° 8.328' W86° 50.490'

From Exit 1 on I-440, south of downtown Nashville, take West End Avenue west 1.6 miles to turn right on Cherokee Road. Follow Cherokee Road 0.6 mile to turn left into the entrance for McCabe Golf Course (the last bit of this part is on Sloan Road, as Cherokee Road becomes Sloan Road). There is parking immediately on the right after you turn into the golf course entrance. This is known as the McCabe Trailhead.

---

13 Shelby Bottoms Nature Park: East Loop

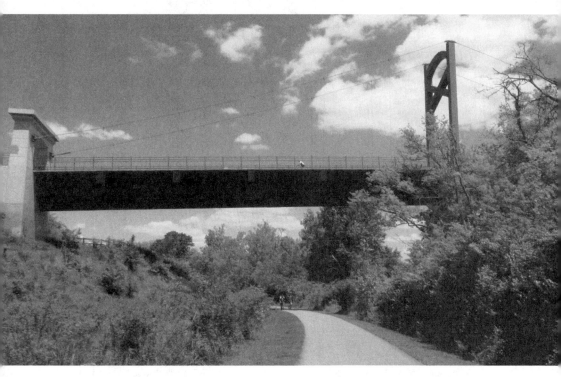

Hiking under the bridge connecting Shelby Bottoms with Stones River Greenway across the Cumberland River

In Brief

The trails of Shelby Bottoms Nature Park were developed from west to east along the banks of the Cumberland River. The nature park offers paved greenways and primitive natural-surface trails. This less traveled East Loop travels both surfaces as it winds among old fields, beneath the foliage of huge trees, in forestland, and by the river where Nashville was founded.

Description

This is a great hike for a crisp day during the cooler season. Much of the trail is in the open, which makes it prohibitively hot during summer. A weak winter sun, on the other hand, casting long shadows across fields and through barren trees, provides the best

Shelby Bottoms Nature Park: East Loop

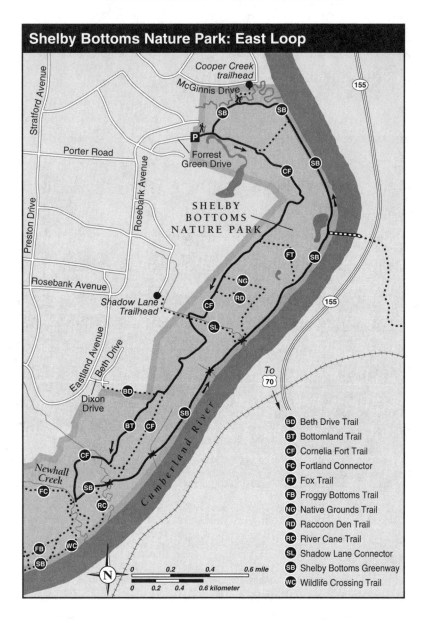

Legend:

- BD Beth Drive Trail
- BT Bottomland Trail
- CF Cornelia Fort Trail
- FC Fortland Connector
- FT Fox Trail
- FB Froggy Bottoms Trail
- NG Native Grounds Trail
- RD Raccoon Den Trail
- RC River Cane Trail
- SL Shadow Lane Connector
- SB Shelby Bottoms Greenway
- WC Wildlife Crossing Trail

atmosphere at this nature park. The fields in this often flooded bottomland were once tilled for crops, just as aborigines did long before Nashville ever existed. Today, the park is being managed for wildlife. You will notice that many of the old fields are being allowed to revert to forest, and the transition is in many different stages. Patches of woodland are interspersed among the fields, most often along streambeds. Also scattered among the bottoms are large trees, which undoubtedly shaded the old farm buildings.

Leave the trailside kiosk after looking at the map. Various loop hikes are plentiful, but the following loop takes you through the most diverse terrain on the eastern side. Be

DISTANCE AND CONFIGURATION: 5.2-mile loop	**ACCESS:** No fees or permits required
DIFFICULTY: Easy	**PETS:** On leash only
SCENERY: Fields, woods, riverside	**MAPS:** USGS *Nashville East;* at **greenwaysfornashville.org/maps-trails /sm_files/shelby%202014.pdf**
EXPOSURE: Mostly sunny	
TRAFFIC: Quiet on weekdays, busy on weekends	**FACILITIES:** Water fountain at trailhead
TRAIL SURFACE: Asphalt, grass, dirt	**CONTACT:** 615-862-8539; **tinyurl.com/shelbybottomsnc**
HIKING TIME: 2.6 hours	**LOCATION:** Nashville

apprised that most trail junctions are not marked, so pay close attention to avoid wandering around without knowing where you are.

Leave the Forrest Green trailhead, and soon you'll intersect the Shelby Bottoms Greenway coming in from your left; this will be your return route. Stay straight on an asphalt track, passing a sometimes flooded wetland on your right. The terrain is mostly open as you keep along a wooded strip that was once a fence line. At 0.2 mile, turn right onto the gravel Cornelia Fort Trail, which soon loses its gravel and cruises along the old fence line. Ahead, you'll pass under two of the biggest hackberry trees in Middle Tennessee. Then curve right, where you'll see other old-growth trees in the area—chestnut, oak, and beech. Cut through a low, wooded area, and then climb to a field broken by occasional strips of woodland that shade intermittent streambeds. The former Cornelia Fort Airport, now part of the park, is visible to your right.

As Fox Trail turns left, keep straight in young trees. Watch for Native Grounds Trail, then Raccoon Den Trail veering off to the left. Continue on Cornelia Fort Trail as it turns right, then left, passing over a small, clear stream to meet Shadow Lane Connector at mile 1.3. This paved greenway heads left to meet Shelby Bottoms Greenway and right to Shadow Lane. You, however, continue on the Cornelia Fort Trail, crossing the paved greenway, and then veer left toward a bank of trees.

Now on the natural-surface Cornelia Fort Trail, you'll come alongside a tree bank and bisect a strip of woodland to reach a trail junction. Turn right onto Bottomland Trail and enter a rich hardwood forest of sweetgum, oak, and hackberry. Stay left where Beth Drive Trail leads to an adjacent neighborhood, and enjoy a woodland walk. Ahead on the left is a monstrous beech tree. Here, Beech Trail intersects Cornelia Fort Trail. Turn right and pass over a low, wet area rife with bamboo before emerging into open field and reaching Shelby Bottoms Greenway at mile 2.4. Turn left on the paved path and begin the return leg of the loop. If you want, take River Cane Trail for extra mileage.

You'll enter woodland and span a gullied streambed. The Cumberland River is to your right as the trail follows the wooded riverbank. Shortly bridge two more streambeds before again intersecting Shadow Lane Connector. Shelby Bottoms Greenway descends to span another streambed on an iron trestle bridge. The trailside becomes more wooded, and Native Grounds Trail soon enters from the left. You stay on paved pathway, though. Dense stands of cane line the trail at times.

Soon you'll intersect Fox Trail, but stay on the greenway and pass under the Cumberland River pedestrian bridge, which connects Shelby Bottoms to Stones River Greenway. Wooded rock bluffs are visible on the far side of the Cumberland. The greenway bends north with the river as fields open to your left. At mile 4.7, a paved path—part of a short loop from the Forrest Green trailhead—leaves left. Keep forward, curving left along Cooper Creek and leaving the Cumberland. Ahead, a bridge spans Cooper Creek to an alternate trailhead off McGinnis Drive. Shelby Bottoms Greenway shortly reaches the trail junction beside the trailhead. Turn right, walk a few steps, and complete the loop.

Nearby Activities

Nearby Shelby Park offers a nature center, fishing, ball fields, tennis courts, and picnic grounds. The west side of Shelby Bottoms Nature Park also has trails.

GPS TRAILHEAD COORDINATES
N36° 11.783' W86° 42.187'

From I-40 just east of downtown Nashville, take Exit 211B; head west on I-24 to Exit 47A (US 31E North/Ellington Parkway/Spring Street). Stay right beyond the interstate, following Ellington Parkway. In 0.7 mile, exit Ellington Parkway onto Cleveland Street. Turn right on Cleveland Street, which becomes Eastland Avenue. Stay on Cleveland/Eastland 0.6 mile; turn left on Gallatin Avenue. Follow Gallatin Avenue 1 mile to Cahal Avenue. Turn right on Cahal and follow it 1 mile, continuing as Cahal becomes Porter Road. Go 1 mile farther on Porter and intersect Rosebank Avenue. Turn left on Rosebank Avenue and soon turn right on Welcome Lane. Head just a short way on Welcome Lane, and then turn left on Forrest Green Drive to soon dead-end at the trailhead.

14 Shelby Bottoms Nature Park: West Loop

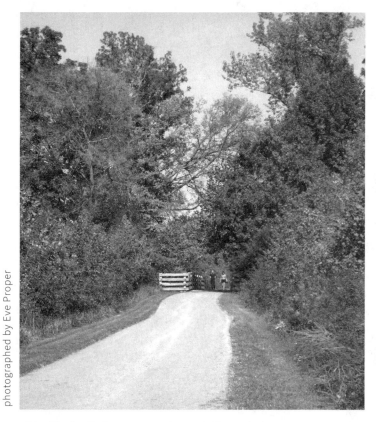

The Shelby Bottoms greenway cuts through dense riverside woods.

In Brief

Shelby Bottoms Nature Park, located on the banks of the Cumberland River just 3 miles from downtown Nashville, is the setting for this hike. Partly on paved greenway and partly on primitive trail, this loop traverses fields, woods, and riverside environments while circling the western edge of the park. Bird lovers will enjoy the walk, as the meadows, wooded edges, and bird boxes enhance avian life. Touch on Nashville history as well, through the trailside interpretive information.

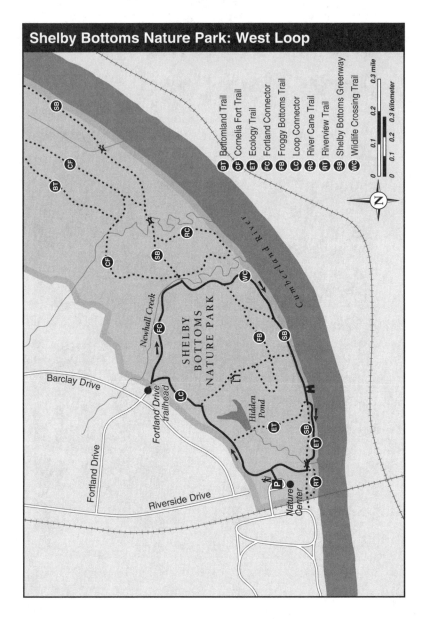

Shelby Bottoms Nature Park: West Loop

Description

At first glance, it is hard to believe such a large, level area so close to downtown Nashville is undeveloped. But there is a reason—this riverside agglomeration of fields and woods is simply too close to the Cumberland River, which is always susceptible to flooding. The city of Nashville saw this 810-acre plot adjacent to Shelby Park as not only a valuable addition to the park system but also the absolute best use of the land. So, since 1997, Music City residents have been enjoying the paved and primitive trails that wind through Shelby Bottoms.

DISTANCE AND CONFIGURATION: 1.8-mile loop	**ACCESS:** No fees or permits required
DIFFICULTY: Easy	**PETS:** On leash only
SCENERY: Fields, woods, riparian environment	**MAPS:** USGS *Nashville East;* at **greenwaysfornashville.org/maps-trails /sm_files/shelby%202014.pdf**
EXPOSURE: Mostly sunny	**FACILITIES:** Restrooms, water fountains at adjacent Shelby Park
TRAFFIC: Steady, busy on weekends	
TRAIL SURFACE: Asphalt, grass, mulch, gravel	**CONTACT:** 615-862-8539; **tinyurl.com/shelbybottomsnc**
HIKING TIME: 1 hour	**LOCATION:** Nashville

Leave the parking area and pass a trailside kiosk. Ahead is a wooden bridge over a wetland. (Wetlands are scattered throughout the bottoms and are an important component of the park.) Ahead is a second kiosk with a good map of the bottoms. The trails are plotted on the kiosk map but not signed on the trails themselves.

Turn left on the paved trail leaving from the kiosk. The path is mostly devoid of trees because Shelby Bottoms has been cultivated by Nashvillians for generations. And why not? As the Cumberland River floods, it deposits rich sediment, making the bottoms a fertile place. Aborigines of a thousand years ago realized this and farmed the area's productive soil.

Pass through a strip of woodland. Beyond the strip, some fields are mowed, and others are growing up around you. Notice the young pine, maple, and sycamore trees. One day this path will be completely shaded. But for now, songbirds, deer, and other critters thrive in the edges between the woods and fields. Bird boxes are also scattered along the trail. This path is currently so open overhead that it would not be fun to hike on a hot summer day. And the houses to your left are just above the floodplain and outside the park boundary.

At 0.2 mile, Ecology Trail leaves right. Stay straight on the paved trail, and then leave left on the grassy Loop Connector at 0.4 mile. Ahead, pass a pedestrian access trail leaving left to Fortland Drive; turn right here. Willow trees indicate a marsh, part of greater Newhall Creek, on your left. The combination of marsh on one side of the trail and field on the other makes an excellent avian habitat. Don't be surprised if winged creatures burst forth from the high field grass and flap for the wooded marsh as you pass by.

Turn right onto the paved Shelby Bottoms Greenway, the master path of the nature park and the halfway point. Stay on it briefly, and then turn left onto Wildlife Crossing Trail. The trail is now shaded by a margin of woods along the riverbank. Watch for the side trail leading left to the river and a view of Demonbreun Cave across the Cumberland. This cave is named for the same man for whom the downtown Nashville street is named. Back in 1769, he actually spelled his name De Montbrun, but the spelling became corrupted along the way. Ol' De Montbrun hunted here and used the cave as a refuge from American Indians. And his wife is said to have birthed the first child of European descent in Middle Tennessee in a nearby cave.

Stay on the paved path, passing a paved trail leading right toward an observation deck and Froggy Bottoms Trail. Ahead, reach a pierlike river overlook. The castlelike structure you see in the middle of the river is part of the Nashville Waterworks complex across the river, which provides water for the city's residents. Built in 1892, the structure is a water-intake valve that's no longer functioning.

Leave the paved greenway at an intersection. Head left on Ecology Trail. Overhead are tall sycamore, cottonwood, and hackberry trees. Enjoy the natural environment down here, imagining the area as it was hundreds of years ago.

Soon you'll rejoin the paved greenway, where you'll find an informative board about exotic plants and birds that have helped create the landscape you see today. It makes you realize that the world has changed for good. Cross a bridge over a dry ravine, and then turn right, passing by the trailhead kiosk to complete the loop.

Nearby Activities

Nearby Shelby Park offers a nature center, fishing, ball fields, tennis courts, and picnic grounds. For more information, visit **nashville.gov/Parks-and-Recreation/Parks/Shelby -Park.aspx.**

GPS TRAILHEAD COORDINATES
N36° 9.955' W86° 43.492'

From I-40 just east of downtown Nashville, take Exit 211B. Then head west on I-24 to Exit 49 (Korean Vets Boulevard/Shelby Avenue/L P Field). Head east on Summer Place for just a short distance, and turn right on Fifth Street. Continue on Fifth Street 0.5 mile to Davidson Street. Turn left on Davidson Street and continue 1.3 miles to enter Shelby Bottoms. Drive beyond the ball fields and keep right, making a right turn in another 0.6 mile to pass under elevated railroad tracks. The parking area is just beyond the tracks.

15 South Radnor Lake Loop

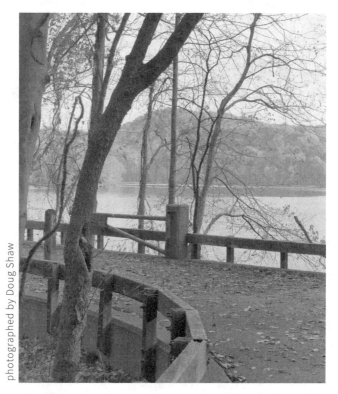

The trail cruises by Radnor Lake.

photographed by Doug Shaw

In Brief

This hike winds through lush north-facing woods on the southern side of Radnor Lake State Park. The forest is rich with wildflowers in spring, is about as cool as the Middle Tennessee outdoors can get in summer, and offers a mosaic of color in fall. In winter, parts of this loop receive very little sun. Don't let the loop's short distance belie its challenging climbs, though.

Description

Get ready for a short but strenuous workout—but first you have to find the trailhead. The South Lake Trailhead is not immediately evident from the visitor center's parking area because it is a good way down Otter Creek Road. Leave the parking area and then walk around the car barriers on Otter Creek Road. Head uphill as the road bridges Otter Creek.

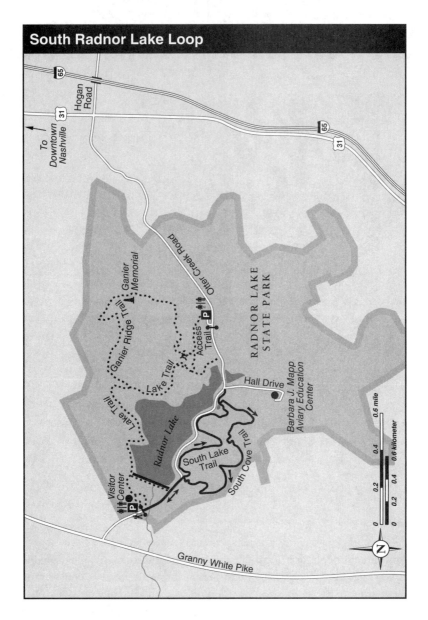

South Radnor Lake Loop

You'll come to Radnor Lake Dam on your left. A side trail leads over the dam. Keep forward, and at 0.2 mile, on a left turn, reach the trailhead on the right side of Otter Creek Road.

Enter the woods, walk a few feet, and turn left on the South Lake Trail. Then begin walking east along the lower slope of a surprisingly steep hill. These are known as the Overton Hills, even though they lie within the town limits of Forest Hills, an enclave now enveloped by the city of Nashville. Travel beneath a hardwood forest of maple and oak, and Radnor Lake, 85 acres in size, is off to your left. This lake was impounded in 1914 by

DISTANCE AND CONFIGURATION: 2.5-mile loop	**ACCESS:** No fees or permits required; daily, 6 a.m.–sunset
DIFFICULTY: Moderate	**PETS:** On leash only
SCENERY: Lush hardwood forest	**MAPS:** USGS *Oak Hill;* at **tnstateparks**
EXPOSURE: Very shady	**.com/parks/about/radnor-lake**
TRAFFIC: Fairly busy, especially on weekends	**FACILITIES:** Restrooms, water at nature center
TRAIL SURFACE: Dirt, rocks	**CONTACT:** 615-373-3467; **tnstateparks .com/parks/about/radnor-lake**
HIKING TIME: 1.5 hours	**LOCATION:** Nashville

the Louisville and Nashville (L&N) Railroad to furnish water for their steam engines and livestock at the nearby, long-disappeared Radnor Yards. This lake initially was a private hunting and fishing preserve for L&N officials. Shortly after the lake was impounded, both native and migratory birds began using the lake. L&N officials realized the natural importance of the lake and declared it a wildlife sanctuary at the request of the Tennessee Ornithological Society.

Ascend the steep hillside. It's so steep, in fact, that wooden berms have been placed on the downside of the trail to keep it level and prevent erosion. Numerous downed trees lie in various states of decay, and it's easy to see the slow but sure cycle of plant life here. It may take a hundred years or more for a tree to grow robust and tall before wind, lightning, or disease strikes it down. Then the tree lies on the ground for decades, slowly rotting and serving as a home and a food source for nature's smaller critters and bugs. But the very richness of the decay will someday feed another tree growing in its place. And so the cycle goes, extending through many human lifetimes.

Work back down toward Radnor Lake along a dry drainage area, passing some sizable oaks. Also notice the deeply fissured trunks of locust trees. These pioneer trees grow in disturbed or cleared areas. The short-lived locust grows rapidly and provides shade for less-sun-tolerant trees, such as sugar maple, then falls and provides nutrients for the trees that follow.

Ahead, a small pond filled with bright-green duck moss lies between the hillside and Otter Creek Road. Circle around the pond, as a side trail leads down to Otter Creek Road. Soon you'll reach a trail junction at mile 1. South Lake Trail keeps straight, but you turn right and take South Cove Trail. Immediately head up a tough hill, and then swing around a cove. In this area the woods are tangled with vines.

Bridge a ravine and begin switchbacking up a hill, meeting an old woods road at some wide steps. Soon top out on the ridgeline, with its obscured views to the north and south at mile 1.6. The trail splits here. To the left, the old road heads a short distance to one of the many contemplation benches set along the path. The main trail swings around a rib ridge with shagbark hickories and thick ground cover. Return shortly to the main ridgeline. Then descend on the old woods road into a tangle of thick woods in the heart of

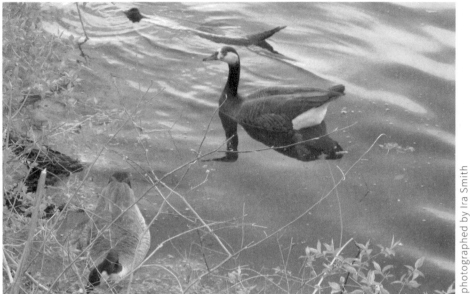

Geese along the shore of Radnor Lake

photographed by Ira Smith

a cove that sees very little sun. You'll soon meet the South Lake Trail. Walk a few feet to Otter Creek Road and backtrack to the visitor center.

Nearby Activities

Be sure to stop at the visitor center before or after this hike. It offers an excellent movie about saving the park as well as other nature displays.

GPS TRAILHEAD COORDINATES
N36° 3.745' W86° 48.597'

From Exit 78 on I-65, south of downtown Nashville, take TN 255/Harding Place west 2.2 miles to Granny White Pike; along the way, Harding Place becomes Battery Lane. Turn left on Granny White Pike and follow it 1.7 miles to Otter Creek Road. Turn left on Otter Creek Road and drive 0.3 mile to the parking area on the left. South Lake Trail starts 0.2 mile down the closed portion of Otter Creek Road beyond the parking area.

16 Stones River Greenway of Nashville

In Brief

Murfreesboro developed the first greenway along the Stones River, but Nashville is giving them a run for their money with this scenic gem that begins just below J. Percy Priest Dam and runs along the Stones in a real mix of attractive settings. The trail stretches a full 10 miles, linking to Shelby Bottoms via pedestrian bridge over the Cumberland River.

Description

Like most who've visited this area, I have driven I-40 past J. Percy Priest Dam and have seen the large flat and spillway next to the interstate. It's easy to tell by the many cars parked there that fishing is popular. But upon taking the Stones River Greenway, which follows the once again free-flowing Stones River, I realized it's also a great place to take a walk.

The track, about 8 feet wide and paved, heads away from the dam. Before leaving the area, though, you may want to check out the fishermen trying their best to get a lunker out of the dam spillway, where the Stones River is once again free to flow to meet the Cumberland River. Pass underneath the double bridges of I-40, and you'll soon leave the noise behind. Because the Stones River flows from the bottom of the lake through the dam, it is normally clear, green, and cold. Notice attractive bluffs across the river and a wooden fence that stands between the river and the greenway.

Even when the greenway doesn't border the river, short gravel-and-dirt tracks lead to the water's edge. At 0.5 mile, a paved path leads left and uphill to an adjoining neighborhood. And at 0.7 mile, the path reaches a particularly scenic area. Here, the path bridges McCrory Creek, a beautiful blue stream that still exemplifies the coloration of many creeks in Middle Tennessee. Here, the slow waters wind to meet the Stones River. A path leads right to a hilly overlook of McCrory Creek and onward to the actual confluence of McCrory Creek and the Stones River. Take the time to explore this little locale.

Continue beyond the bridge, and the trail opens to a field. Here, a parallel track runs through the grassland, and the greenway turns to dip into fully shaded thick woods along the Stones River. Notice the large sycamores along the river. At 1 mile, the trail passes two concrete structures that I believe were water-gauging stations. The trail then reenters a field and continues downstream to span a smaller branch on a steel truss bridge at 1.4 miles. The creek here cuts a steep, deep valley for its size. Just ahead, you can see the cut-stone abutments of an old bridge spanning the Stones River. A dirt track leading right heads to the base of one abutment and allows you to see another abutment standing silently in the river. You'll notice a cedar tree growing from the top of this pillar.

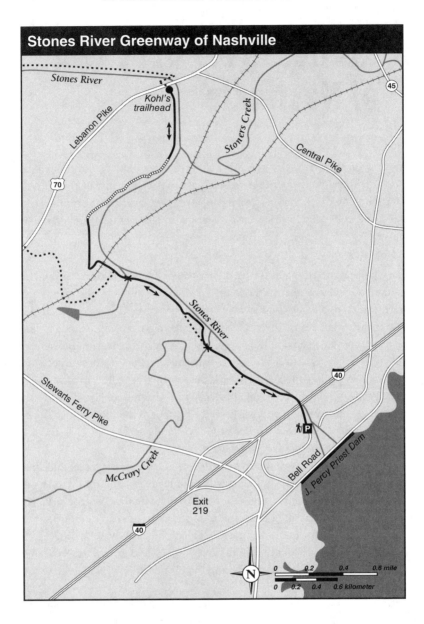

Stones River Greenway of Nashville

The greenway passes under a railroad bridge before making its big climb, and the path turns uphill to reach the top of a bluff over the river. Top out at 1.8 miles and pass under some power lines before descending to the river and the highlight of the greenway. After skirting the edge of some condos, the greenway works its way downstream along a boardwalk that parallels the river bluffs. From this boardwalk, walkers have great views up and down the Stones.

DISTANCE AND CONFIGURATION: 6-mile out-and-back	**PETS:** On leash only
DIFFICULTY: Moderate	**MAPS:** USGS *Hermitage* and USGS *Nashville East;* at **greenwaysfornashville.org**
SCENERY: Woods, fields, riverside	**/PDFmaps/StonesRiver.pdf**
EXPOSURE: Part sun, part shade	**FACILITIES:** Restrooms and picnic area at nearby J. Percy Priest Dam Army Corps of Engineers visitor center
TRAFFIC: Moderate to heavy on weekends	
TRAIL SURFACE: Paved	**CONTACT:** 615-862-8400; **nashville.gov/Parks-and-Recreation**
HIKING TIME: 2.5 hours	
ACCESS: No fees or permits required	**LOCATION:** Nashville

The boardwalk rejoins terra firma at 2.2 miles, and the greenway keeps near the Stones, crossing intermittent streambeds west of the river. Near Lebanon Pike, the trail turns uphill to reach what is commonly called the Kohl's trailhead, ending at 2.9 miles. This trailhead is in a shopping center parking lot near the Kohl's store off Lebanon Pike, east of Briley Parkway. Most greenway users simply backtrack to the dam trailhead. The greenway continues onward to border the Cumberland River near its confluence with the Stones at Heartland Park, where there is a trailhead. Another trailhead is located at Two Rivers Park. After curving near the Wave Country attraction, a pedestrian bridge across the Cumberland River links Shelby Bottoms Greenway to the Stones River Greenway.

Nearby Activities

J. Percy Priest Dam has fishing, picnicking, and all the pleasures of a big lake behind it. Stones River makes for a fine 7-mile canoe or kayak trip to the Cumberland River with a takeout at Peeler Park boat ramp. For information about the dam area, the put-in for a Stones River paddling trip, visit the Army Corps of Engineers website at **www.lrn.usace .army.mil/Locations/Dams/JPercyPriestDam.aspx.**

GPS TRAILHEAD COORDINATES
N36° 9.473' W86° 37.233'

From Exit 219 on I-40, east of downtown Nashville, take Stewarts Ferry Pike south 0.2 mile to Bell Road. Turn left on Bell Road and follow it to an intersection. The right turn is into the J. Percy Priest Dam visitor center. Take the left turn at this intersection, dropping down to a large, level area below the dam. Stones River Greenway begins at the northern end of the parking area, toward I-40.

17 Volunteer-Day Loop

In Brief

This hike explores the wilder side of Long Hunter State Park. Follow Volunteer Trail 0.5 mile through the woods and pick up the Day Loop Trail, which skirts the rocky shoreline of J. Percy Priest Lake. Circle around to a high bluff and enjoy stunning lake views before reaching a quiet cove that was once settled. Ramble over a hill filled with tall oaks, and then backtrack 0.5 mile to finish the hike.

Description

The state of Tennessee is fortunate to be in control of this parkland that covers some 33 shoreline miles of J. Percy Priest Lake. As Nashville has expanded and lakeshore property has become more desirable for housing, the value of this land has skyrocketed. In fact, to obtain this shoreline now would break the state's budget. The property is currently under a 99-year lease from the U.S. Army Corps of Engineers, which dammed J. Percy Priest Lake in 1968. Long Hunter State Park was established shortly after the damming.

And how pretty this trail is, running along the shore, over limestone outcrops, through streamsheds, and around peninsulas jutting into the lake. Start your hike on the white-blazed Volunteer Trail, named for Boy Scout volunteers who constructed the path. Walk down an old gravel road flanked with brush. Off to your right is an overgrown fence line, and the sky is open overhead. Soon you'll leave the roadbed and turn right into a forest carpeted with *Vinca minor,* also known as cemetery ivy. Not surprisingly, this was once a burial place. The Corps of Engineers relocated the cemetery when the dam was built. You'll pass a small sinkhole to the right of the trail. Keep forward to reach a footbridge with handrails; it spans a wet-weather drainage area that forms the lake cove visible to your left.

The path picks and twists its way amid a rock jumble before reaching a junction at 0.6 mile. Turn left on the orange-blazed Day Loop Trail, immediately stepping over a dry wash. Stay along the shoreline in a young forest. The trail here runs alongside a limestone rampart running parallel to the shoreline, zigzagging through the rocks, sometimes above the rampart, sometimes below. At mile 1, the path nears J. Percy Priest Lake. Walk a few feet to the shoreline.

You are now looking over the Stones River valley, which was flooded to create J. Percy Priest Lake. The Stones River was named for Uriah Stone, a long hunter of yesteryear. When explorers, settlers, and hunters began pouring westward over the Appalachian Mountains in the mid-1700s, some of them would explore the fringes of settled land and American Indian territory for extended periods that became known as long hunts. During periods lasting up to a year, the hunters would acquire hides and furs of deer, beaver, elk, and otters, then return east to sell them. These men, who made their living in the fur trade, became known as long hunters.

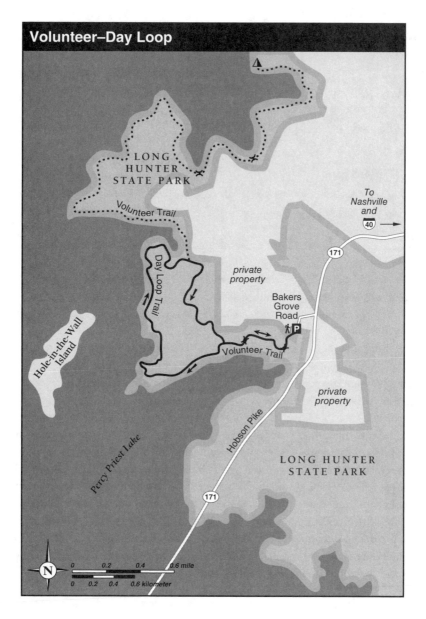

Uriah Stone favored the hunting grounds of a particular river heading south from the Cumberland River. On one trip near this river, he was double-crossed by a Frenchman with whom he had partnered, who stole his hides. Other long hunters named the Stones River after him as a result of this episode. Consequently, 200 years later, Long Hunter State Park was named for the Stones River valley that it abuts.

DISTANCE AND CONFIGURATION: 4-mile loop	**MAPS:** USGS *La Vergne;* at **tinyurl.com/longhuntermap**
DIFFICULTY: Moderate	**FACILITIES:** None
SCENERY: Hardwood and cedar forest, rock bluffs, lake views	**CONTACT:** 615-885-2422; **tnstateparks .com/parks/about/long-hunter**
EXPOSURE: Nearly all shady	**LOCATION:** Hermitage
TRAFFIC: Busy on weekends	**COMMENTS:** Volunteer Trail continues to a backcountry campsite. The Bakers Grove Recreation Area part of Long Hunter State Park is primitive, but the Couchville Unit of the state park has a visitor center, pic- nic area, rental canoes, and more trails.
TRAIL SURFACE: Dirt, rocks, leaves	
HIKING TIME: 2.1 hours	
ACCESS: No fees or permits required	
PETS: On leash only	

Turn away from the lake at mile 1.1 and notice small sinks and rock outcrops amid the thick woodland area. The trail makes a sharp U-turn near an old fence line, then returns to the lake's edge. Here, you can look west across the lake at a rock bluff on Hole-in-the-Wall Island. To your right, in the distance, is the shoreline along which the Volunteer Trail continues to a backcountry campsite. Cruise along the shoreline and soon you'll reach a small pond separated from the lake by only a thin strip of trees.

The shoreline steepens and the trail climbs, reaching a bluffline that offers dramatic views. Watch your step here among the rocks. Eventually leave the bluffline and head farther inland. Turn away from the lake, ascending alongside a deep, dry creek bed. Piles of rocks indicate that this area may have been farmed at one time. Turn back downstream on the dry creek bed and intersect the Volunteer Trail at a second dry drainage at mile 2.7. Just across the drainage, to the left, are an information board and the trek to the back-country campsite. Turn right on the Volunteer Trail, begin climbing along this drainage, and pass an old stone fence at mile 2.8. Keep ascending over a wooded hill. Make a hard right at mile 3.1, briefly picking up an old woods road. Soon turn left off the old road to make a prolonged descent along a streambed. Cross this streambed to reach a familiar junction at mile 3.4. Stay forward, as the Day Loop Trail you already hiked leaves right, and retrace your steps 0.6 mile to the trailhead.

GPS TRAILHEAD COORDINATES
N36° 6.185' W86° 33.152'

From Exit 226 on I-40, east of downtown Nashville, take TN 171/South Mount Juliet Road 4.2 miles south. Veer right at the split as TN 171 becomes Hobson Pike. Continue 1.8 miles farther, turning right on Bakers Grove Lane. Drive just a short distance; then turn left on Bakers Grove Road and follow it a short distance to the parking area at the dead end.

18 Warner Woods Trail

In Brief

Big trees, deep woods, and a good view are all rolled into one hike located less than 10 air miles from downtown Nashville. This loop hike traverses land set aside by Luke Lea for a park near the town of Belle Meade, now enveloped by greater Nashville. Hikers will pass several large, old-growth trees amid a rich forest and Luke Lea Heights, which offers a far-reaching view of the Nashville Basin, downtown Nashville, and beyond.

Description

While on your hike, you might want to thank Percy Warner, who was chairman of the Nashville Park Board in the 1920s. Warner's son-in-law, Luke Lea, was in the process of developing what would later become the town of Belle Meade when Warner convinced Lea to donate some of his land for this park. Warner died suddenly after this deal was made, and the park was named for him. Adjacent Edwin Warner Park is named for Warner's brother, who became the next park-board chairman. Currently these two parks total 2,684 acres, 2,058 of which are in Percy Warner Park.

Begin Warner Woods Trail behind the covered trail-map kiosk, and trace the white-blazed path to immediately cross Old Beech bridle path. Continue, climbing a hill, and reach another junction. Here the red-blazed Mossy Ridge Trail goes right, and the white-blazed Warner Woods Trail goes left. Turn left, looking up on the hillside to your right beyond the junction for a giant white oak. Soon cross the Deep Well Cut Off bridle path. Continue, passing a huge tulip tree, and reach the loop portion of Warner Woods Trail. Turn left and begin to swing around a knob of the Harpeth Hills, climbing through rich, vine-draped woods to reach Farrell Road.

Actually a remnant of the scenic driving roads that course through this park, Farrell Road was never paved, as the remaining scenic roads are today, and has reverted to a rough dirt path. Maples and tulip trees are reclaiming the margins of the way, further diminishing its appearance as a road. Another notable tree in the area is the shagbark hickory, which has an easily identifiable bark that appears to be peeling.

At 0.8 mile, you'll cross a paved scenic road and enter Buggy Bottoms. An intermittent stream sometimes flows here to feed Willow Pond, the body of water beside TN 100. Pass a contemplation bench looking over the remains of a big white oak that is but a skeleton of its former self. Its limbs are slowly falling off, but it will be beyond our lifetimes before this giant has completely returned to the earth. Come alongside a second contemplation bench in Buggy Bottoms adjacent to the intermittent streambed; many exotic vines cling to the trunks of the trees here. Cross the bridle path again and a paved road at mile 1.7. Not far from here, a side trail leads left down to the palatial main entrance to Percy Warner Park at the end of Belle Meade Boulevard.

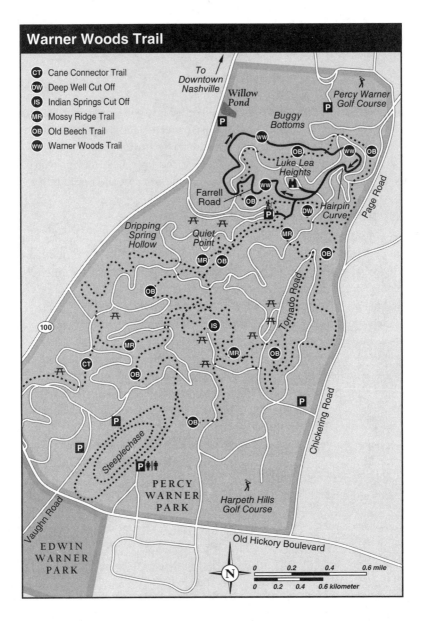

Warner Woods Trail

- **CT** Cane Connector Trail
- **DW** Deep Well Cut Off
- **IS** Indian Springs Cut Off
- **MR** Mossy Ridge Trail
- **OB** Old Beech Trail
- **WW** Warner Woods Trail

The trail then climbs a bit to Hairpin Curve, so named for a turn in the scenic road the trail nears. The crumbled stone wall along the road is evidence that at least one auto didn't make the curve. Warner Woods Trail curves a lot less than the road and keeps ascending toward Luke Lea Heights, reaching a paved road at mile 2.1. Turn right and walk about 50 yards, where the road splits. Look for the foot trail between the two roads that leads straight up the ridgeline. Take this path to shortly emerge at Luke Lea Summit, where a view to the northeast opens up beside a couple of cedar benches. Look to the

DISTANCE AND CONFIGURATION: 2.5-mile loop	**PETS:** On leash only
DIFFICULTY: Easy–moderate	**MAPS:** USGS *Bellevue;* at **tinyurl.com/mossyridgetrl**
SCENERY: Rich hillside woods and views	
EXPOSURE: Shady	**FACILITIES:** Portable bathroom at trailhead
TRAFFIC: Moderate, somewhat busy on weekends	**CONTACT:** 615-352-6299; **tinyurl.com/warnerparknc**
TRAIL SURFACE: Dirt, roots	
HIKING TIME: A little more than an hour	**LOCATION:** Nashville
ACCESS: No fees or permits required; daily, sunrise–11 p.m.	**COMMENTS:** Stay with the white blazes, as there are many trail junctions.

horizon at downtown Nashville and beyond across the Nashville Basin. This 920-foot knob offers an impressive view of downtown Nashville, which lies at about 400 feet in elevation. Backtrack to where Warner Woods Trail crossed the scenic drive, and head downhill, reaching the end of the trail's loop portion at 2.4 miles. From this point, backtrack 0.1 mile to the Deep Well trailhead.

Nearby Activities

The Deep Well Picnic Area has many fine picnic shelters, so consider combining a cookout or outdoor lunch with your hike. For more information, call 615-352-6299 or visit **nashville.gov/parks/wpnc**.

GPS TRAILHEAD COORDINATES

N36° 4.703' W86° 52.790'

From the point where TN 100 begins at US 70 near the Belle Meade Post Office, head west on TN 100 for 1.7 miles to the large stone gates on the left that mark the Deep Well entrance of Percy Warner Park. Turn left from TN 100 and pass through the gates, staying right when the road splits. Reach the Deep Well trailhead parking at 0.6 mile. Warner Woods Trail starts behind the trailside kiosk.

WEST

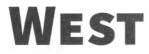

INCLUDING ASHLAND CITY, CLARKSVILLE, AND DICKSON

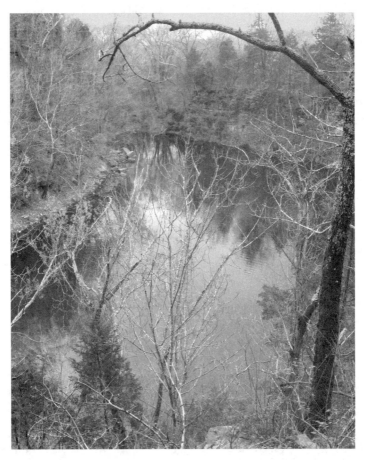

Gazing into Hidden Lake from a waterside bluff (see page 93)

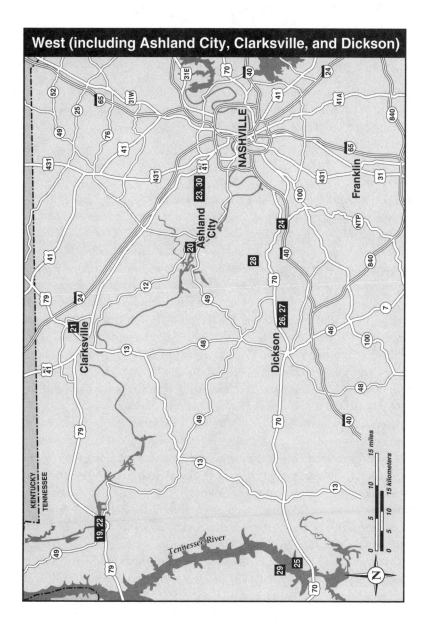

West (including Ashland City, Clarksville, and Dickson)

19 Confederate Earthworks Walk

In Brief

This little-used, underrated path at Fort Donelson National Battlefield traverses a corridor of protected land. In addition to running parallel to Confederate earthworks nearly its entire distance, this trail passes over three sizable hills that were artillery batteries connected by these earthworks.

Description

This trail is so little used that it doesn't even have a name. It could be called Corridor Trail, as it runs east along a narrow strip of land that extends from the preserved Fort Donelson National Battlefield. And it could be called Hill Trail, as it starts atop one hill, then alternately dives and climbs two more hills. But the trail shall remain nameless and languish in solitude, while the nearby primary trails of Fort Donelson get more traffic. (See page 86.)

If you tour Fort Donelson, also take the time to hike this path. It needs some feet on it, and hikers may spot deer as well. Before you hike it, though, stop at the visitor center and get acquainted with the battle that was fought here. Fort Donelson and nearby Fort Henry were built by the Confederate Army to hold sway over the Tennessee and Cumberland Rivers, thwarting the Union Army's efforts to use these waterways for troop or supply movements. Fort Henry was poorly located in a low area subject to flooding by the Tennessee River, and in February 1862 was easily bombed into submission by federal ironclad gunboats. But the rebels escaped east to Fort Donelson, securely located on a hill with a sweeping view of the Cumberland River. The soldiers of Fort Henry reached Fort Donelson, which was already protected by earthworks, then built an outer perimeter of trenches beyond the fort. These earthworks were stretched along high ground from Hickman Creek in the west to the tiny town of Dover in the east. The earthworks you follow on this hike were part of the outer perimeter.

Federal gunboats couldn't do much against the well-placed rebel artillery at Fort Donelson, but while the water war was going on, federal troops amassed around the whole rebel perimeter. The Union crashed the perimeter, but the rebels pushed them back. In the confusion of battle, the rebels were ordered to return to their original positions behind the earthworks. The Union attacked again, retaking territory they had lost and gaining some, to boot. Finally, most of the Confederate soldiers escaped southeast to Nashville, leaving too few to defend Fort Donelson, which was surrendered to Union General Ulysses S. Grant the next day.

While you're hiking, imagine Confederate and Union troops poised on either side of the earthworks beside you. Leave the circular parking area and head downhill on the grassy part

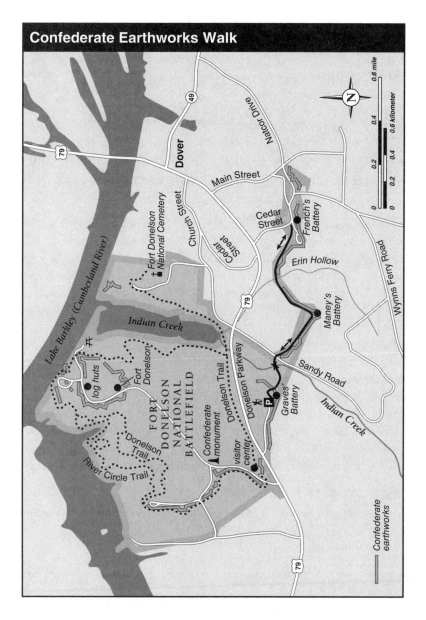

Confederate Earthworks Walk

of the corridor. A cannon representing Graves' Battery is to your right, and a small brown hiker sign leads the way downhill. The mowed field is cut a little lower along the barely discernible trail. Dive off the hill to reach a wooded flat on your left, and the earthworks will be to your right. Cross a quaint little bridge that passes over a clear stream named Indian Creek. Keep forward beyond the bridge through a field flanked on the left by cedar trees.

Reach Sandy Road and continue forward; an interpretive sign about the activities of Nathan Bedford Forrest stands to your left. Then ascend the wooded hill ahead of you. It

DISTANCE AND CONFIGURATION: 2.6-mile out-and-back	**ACCESS:** No fees or permits required
DIFFICULTY: Moderate	**PETS:** Must be leashed on park roads and trails
SCENERY: Forest and field	**MAPS:** USGS *Dover;* at **nps.gov/fodo**
EXPOSURE: Mostly shady, some sun	**FACILITIES:** Restrooms, water at visitor center
TRAFFIC: Very little	
TRAIL SURFACE: Grass, leaves	**CONTACT:** 931-232-0834; **nps.gov/fodo**
HIKING TIME: 1.7 hours	**LOCATION:** Dover

is easy to see the narrowness of this protected corridor as houses are visible nearby. Tall cedar and oak trees shade the route, and the earthworks remain to your right. Continue up the steep hill and top out at the location of Maney's Battery. It is easy to see why the rebel army picked this hilltop with its potential views. Trees were felled back then to open points of observation and clear lines of fire. This four-cannon unit was placed here, along with French's Battery on the next hill, to keep the Union from sneaking down Erin Hollow, where you are headed, and attacking Fort Donelson.

Turn left at Maney's Battery, now descending, again, a long hill. The rebel trenches remain to your right. Shortly you'll arrive at the bottom of Erin Hollow and span the intermittent stream on a wooden bridge. The trail here becomes a bit obscure. Begin climbing uphill, keeping the earthworks to your right.

The trail opens in a field and climbs steeply to the third hill, on top of which is a most attractive setting. Large hardwoods flank a level, grassy area, the site of French's Battery (interpretive signs relate the site's history). Ahead are a small parking area, Cedar Street, and the end of this hike. Retrace your steps through the hills and hollows back to Graves' Battery.

Nearby Activities

Fort Donelson National Battlefield has an informative museum, an auto tour, and a nice picnic area.

GPS TRAILHEAD COORDINATES
N36° 28.891' W87° 51.463'

From Exit 11 on I-24, northwest of downtown Nashville, take TN 76 for 3.4 miles west to a traffic light in Clarksville. TN 76 then becomes US 41A North. Continue on US 41A North 7.9 miles to US 79. Turn left on US 79 South and follow it 31.4 miles to reach Fort Donelson National Battlefield, just past the town of Dover, on your right. Stop at the visitor center and obtain a park map. Drive out of the visitor center and turn left on US 79, heading 0.1 mile back toward Dover. Turn right onto an unnamed paved road and follow it a short distance to dead-end at the location of Graves' Battery. The trail follows the field downhill as you look toward the cannon at Graves' Battery.

20 Cumberland River Bicentennial Trail

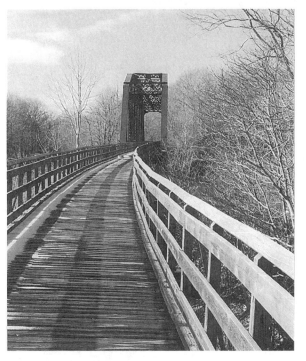

A curved trestle spans Sycamore Creek.

In Brief

This rustic rail-trail quietly runs through a rural section of the lower Cumberland River. The path is flanked by bluffs on one side and water on the other. Look for wildlife.

Description

Ashland City did the right thing by converting the old tracks of the Tennessee Central Railroad into a path that is now enjoyed by nature lovers of all stripes. The valley of the Cumberland River is wide at the point along which the rail-trail travels. To prevent its tracks from flooding, the railroad had built a right-of-way along the northern edge of the river valley. Steep bluffs to the north and a vast floodplain to the south border the trail. The Cumberland River is just out of sight, but the embayment of Sycamore Creek, which

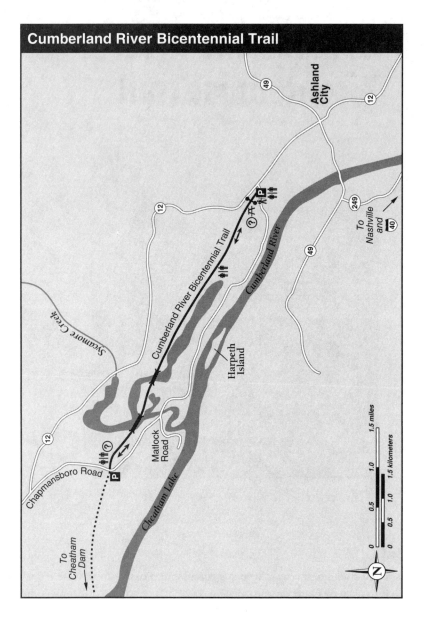

Cumberland River Bicentennial Trail

flows into the Cumberland, lies along much of the rail-trail, lending a watery aspect. Cheatham Dam, downstream on the Cumberland, creates the embayment.

The railroad-turned-greenway passes over small creeks that have cut their way through the riverside bluffs. Here, trestles bridge the creeks, offering a bird's-eye view of the surroundings. In places, the right-of-way has been elevated to keep the former tracks level. The path's flatness makes it appealing for those who want to concentrate on seeing the sights around them, rather than huffing and puffing through hills.

DISTANCE AND CONFIGURATION: 8-mile out-and-back	**ACCESS:** No fees or permits required
DIFFICULTY: Moderate	**PETS:** On leash only
SCENERY: Hardwood forest, creek embayment, small creeks	**MAPS:** USGS *Ashland City;* at **cumberlandrivertrail.org**
EXPOSURE: Mostly shady	**FACILITIES:** Restrooms and picnic tables at trailhead and along the way
TRAFFIC: Some on weekends, but not too busy	**CONTACT:** 615-792-2655; **cumberlandrivertrail.org**
TRAIL SURFACE: Pea gravel, grass, rocks, asphalt	**LOCATION:** Ashland City
HIKING TIME: 3.5 hours	**COMMENTS:** The rail-trail extends beyond this segment.

Start by walking around a metal gate, and immediately you'll pass a trailside kiosk and picnic table. A hardwood forest of sycamore, oak, and sweetgum trees shades the path. Look for railroad ties and occasional steel rails near the greenway, where you'll notice informative signs pointing out specific bushes and wildflowers that bloom along the path in spring. In some places, the yellow-tan bluffs to the right of the trail were blasted to make room for the tracks; cedar trees hang precariously from atop these bluffs. In other places, small creeks have cut through the bluffs and formed little valleys; their waters flow clear below the trail through culverts.

A wooded swamp lies to the left of the trail; farther on, this watery area becomes a full-fledged lake. At mile 1.1, reach the Turkey Junction native gardens and comfort station. To the left are a restroom and a garden encircled by a gravel path. Wastewater flows from the comfort station through a wetland-water-treatment-demonstration system. A signboard explains how the water treatment system works.

Cumberland River Bicentennial Trail continues northwest, passing a second trestle over a small creek at mile 1.4. Here, a side trail leads left to picnic tables beside the Sycamore Creek embayment. The trail straddles the right-of-way between the lake on the left and the bluff on the right, passing a third trestle at mile 1.8. Pass a longer trestle at mile 2.2.

The tree canopy opens by mile 2.4 as an old roadbed goes to the right up a hollow. Soon you'll reach a bridge that stretches 200 feet in length above the embayment and see farm country—old wooden outbuildings, fields, rows of trees—around you. Hills rise on the far side of the Cumberland River. The trailside bluff gives way beyond this last bridge, giving the greenway a more open feel.

At mile 3.2, you'll reach the trestle spanning Sycamore Creek. This trestle is curved and has a steel-frame span in its center; it is by far the largest bridge on the rail-trail. The greenway is paved in asphalt beyond this final bridge. Continue in thick woods and soon you'll reach a trailside kiosk and restroom. Turn right and drop off the elevated right-of-way to reach Chapmansboro Road and the end of this greenway segment. The east side of the road identifies this as the Sycamore Harbor trailhead, and the west side of the road identifies it as the Eagle Pass trailhead. Either way, you have reached the 4-mile mark and the end of this segment. Cheatham Dam is 2.5 miles farther on the greenway.

If you want to hike just 4 miles to this point and not backtrack, use the following directions to the Eagle Pass–Sycamore Harbor trailhead at the other end: Continue past the Marks Creek trailhead on Chapmansboro Road, coming directly alongside the Cumberland River. Bridge the Sycamore Creek embayment 3.4 miles from the Marks Creek trailhead and immediately turn right onto the continuation of Chapmansboro Road. Pass several houses and look left for a parking area 0.9 mile from the Sycamore Creek embayment.

The Cumberland River Bicentennial Trail continues west and now stretches almost 8 continuous miles.

GPS TRAILHEAD COORDINATES

N36° 17.108' W87° 4.707'

From Exit 188 on I-40, west of downtown Nashville, take TN 249 North and drive 16.7 miles to reach TN 49. Turn right onto TN 49 East, and cross the Cumberland River to reach Ashland City and TN 12 in 1 mile. Turn left on TN 12, and follow it north 1.1 miles to Chapmansboro Road. Turn left on Chapmansboro Road, and follow it 0.1 mile to the Marks Creek trailhead on your right.

21 Dunbar Cave State Natural Park Loop

In Brief

This hike uses two park trails to form a loop. It travels in the woods, along Swan Lake and beside the park's namesake Dunbar Cave. If the walk doesn't do enough for your legs, consider adding a cave tour, which follows underground paths.

Description

Let's face it—Dunbar Cave was preserved more for its underground features than those that the sun shines upon. However, its aboveground features are attractive and as worthy of a visit as the cave. The city of Clarksville has grown around Dunbar Cave State Natural Park, creating a suburban park in the process and making the green space it provides even more valuable. These 110 acres are mostly former farmland, complemented by a lake fed by springs flowing from Dunbar Cave.

Your loop hike traverses the Lake Trail and the Recovery Trail, which is named for the surrounding forest that has recovered from clearing. So lace up your boots and come on up for a hike.

Leave the upper parking area and start the Recovery Trail. Picnic tables are scattered around the trailhead. Follow a former road of crumbling pavement that once led to Dunbar Cave, and you'll see Swan Lake down the hill to your right. At 0.1 mile, a side trail leads right to the entrance of Dunbar Cave. You may not be able to squelch your curiosity, so go ahead and walk to the mouth of the cave. It has a cathedral-like opening, though the actual cave entrance is much smaller. It is easy to visualize live band music playing in the cave mouth when country-music legend Roy Acuff owned it. He and others not only held concerts and dances here but also broadcast a live country-music radio program from Dunbar. Before that, in the 1880s, the cave and adjacent springs, now used to fill Swan Lake, were part of a mineral-springs resort. And before that, Tennessee's pre-Columbian American Indians used it for shelter. Upon the arrival of Tennessee's settlers, a fellow named Dunbar bought the land and gave the cave its name. The state of Tennessee purchased and took over the land and its underground treasures in 1972.

Return to the Recovery Trail (the crumbling pavement has given way to natural trail surface), and pass through a cleared area. Just ahead, the Short Loop Trail turns right. The Recovery Trail continues up a hollow and curves right, uphill, through oak woods. Top out in a cedar thicket, drop down the hill, and take the first of three right turns to enter bottomland populated with sycamore trees. The older forest is flanked by a rocky hillside to your right. Wildflowers abound in this bottom during spring.

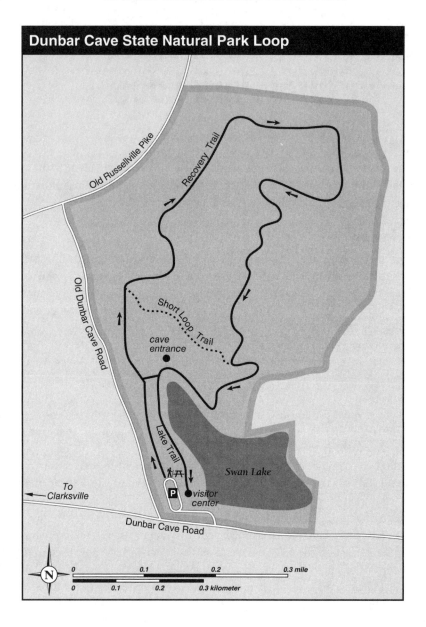

Ascend away from the bottom to meet the Short Loop at mile 1.2, which comes in from the right. Here, the trail once continued, but it has since been rerouted to descend toward Swan Lake in a more snakelike, less erosive route. Turn left at the junction, following the newer Lake Trail as it makes its way to Swan Lake. Large oak trees shade the now paved path along the lake.

The visitor center is visible across the water. This white building was once part of the resort and was converted to park offices and informative displays after being acquired by

DISTANCE AND CONFIGURATION: 1.8-mile loop	**ACCESS:** No fees or permits required
DIFFICULTY: Easy	**PETS:** On 6-foot leash only
SCENERY: Hardwood and cedar forest, lake, cave entrance	**MAPS:** USGS *Clarksville;* at **tnstateparks .com/parks/about/dunbar-cave**
EXPOSURE: Mostly shady	**FACILITIES:** Restrooms, water at visitor center
TRAFFIC: Fairly steady from locals	
TRAIL SURFACE: Leaves, dirt, rocks, pavement	**CONTACT:** 931-648-5526; **tnstateparks .com/parks/about/dunbar-cave**
HIKING TIME: 1.2 hours	**LOCATION:** Clarksville

Tennessee State Parks. Follow the paved path toward the mouth of Dunbar Cave, and you'll reach the columnar concrete addition to the cave mouth; this area may be busy in summer. Beneath you is the spring upwelling that has been flooded by the damming of Swan Lake in 1933. Circle past the cave entrance, still on the lake perimeter. The geese and ducks you'll see here may be looking for handouts because park visitors often feed them. Shortly you'll reach the steps to access the visitor center and the parking area from where you started.

Nearby Activities

Dunbar Cave State Natural Park offers cave tours daily during May, June, and July. Dunbar Cave has 8 miles of explored and surveyed passages that extend about a half mile into the cave, and it maintains a constant 58°F temperature year-round. Groups touring the cave are encouraged to make reservations. Call ahead for exact tour times and fees at 931-648-5526, or visit **tnstateparks.com/parks/about/dunbar-cave.**

GPS TRAILHEAD COORDINATES

N36° 33.032' W87° 18.370'

From Exit 4 on I-24, northwest of downtown Nashville, take US 79 South 4.2 miles to intersect Dunbar Cave Road. Turn left on Dunbar Cave Road and follow it 1.2 miles to Old Dunbar Cave Road. Turn left on Old Dunbar Cave Road and drive just a short distance to the parking-area entrance on your right. Recovery Trail starts at the upper end of the parking area.

22 Fort Donelson Battlefield Loop

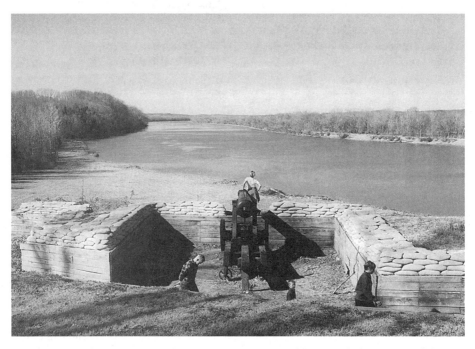

You can see why cannon emplacements were situated here, with this sweep of the Cumberland River.

In Brief

This hike loops the perimeter of Fort Donelson National Battlefield, on the shores of Lake Barkley. Along the way, it visits a monument, river batteries, troop trenches, and log huts from the Civil War. You will be surprised at both the steepness of the terrain and the natural beauty that accompanies this special place.

Description

This is one of Middle Tennessee's great unsung hikes. The historical importance of the trailside location is obvious, but the setting will surprise you. Travel along flanks of Confederate earthworks erected to protect Fort Donelson, which in turn guarded the lower Cumberland River. Pass a tall monument to Confederate soldiers. Then drop to the shores of Lake Barkley to reach Fort Donelson, where river batteries look over a stunning

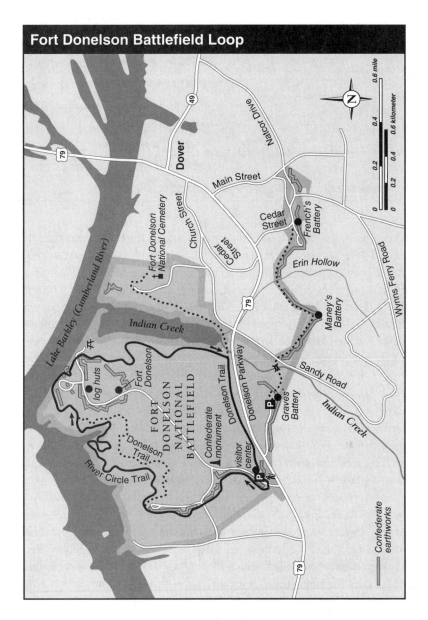

sweep of the Cumberland River. Visit log-hut replicas that housed Confederate troops, and enjoy a woods walk while returning to the visitor center and completing the loop.

To gain an understanding of this battle, which was the first success in the Union's plan to split the Confederacy in two, stop by the visitor center and learn more. In summary, the Confederates fled nearby Fort Henry after being overwhelmed by Union forces. The Union soldiers followed and began surrounding the rebels, who had hastily constructed an outer perimeter of earthworks to protect Fort Donelson. Seeing the futility of

DISTANCE AND CONFIGURATION: 3.3-mile loop	**HIKING TIME:** 2.5 hours
DIFFICULTY: Moderate	**ACCESS:** No fees or permits required
SCENERY: Forests, fields, hardwood ravines, big river	**PETS:** On 6-foot leash at all times
	MAPS: USGS *Dover;* at **nps.gov/fodo**
EXPOSURE: Mostly shady	**FACILITIES:** Restrooms, water at visitor center and picnic area
TRAFFIC: Busy on nice weekends and holidays	**CONTACT:** 931-232-0834; **nps.gov/fodo**
TRAIL SURFACE: Dirt, mulch, grass	**LOCATION:** Dover

their own position, the rebels cleared an escape route up the Cumberland and departed. Others were left to defend the fort and eventually surrendered to Union General Ulysses S. Grant. This battle was the first step from obscurity for the general.

The trail begins near the six-pound cannon, where a sign reads DONELSON TRAIL, 3.1 MILES. In other places the trail is denoted by brown signs with hiker symbols on them. Turn right as you face the sign here, and begin walking a mowed path; Confederate earthworks will be on your right, and the hillside drops steeply to your left. Basically, the earthworks are trenches that protected soldiers. Johnny Reb set up these earthworks, using the steep terrain as an added measure of defense. The Union soldiers had to ascend the hills and storm the trenches to breach this outer perimeter. The setting is attractive with the mixture of scattered trees, grass, and woods.

Shortly, you'll reach the Confederate monument on your right. This tall stone pillar is fronted with a metal Confederate soldier in uniform. Return to the trail and keep north along the rebel trenches, soon passing the site of Union General C. F. Smith's attack and subsequent capture of the earthworks. Ahead is the site of Jackson's Battery, a Confederate position later abandoned when the rebels decided to break for Nashville.

Reach a trail junction at 0.5 mile. Split left onto the River Circle Trail, which soon dives into the Hickman Creek embayment. Cross and follow an intermittent branch to the embayment. Parallel the embayment, then suddenly climb steeply while circling around a ravine. Come near a field; then turn away and drop to a steeply cut hollow. Cross a footbridge over the tiny stream. Just past the footbridge on the right is a rocked-in spring that may have provided water for soldiers during battle.

Pass along the Hickman Creek embayment once more, before intersecting Donelson Trail at mile 1.7. Veer left onto Donelson Trail and soon you'll come out at the Upper River Battery. Here, Confederates used heavy artillery to bombard Union ironclad gunboats into withdrawing. It is easy to see that these well-placed cannons could control the Cumberland River at this point. What you see today is Lake Barkley, formed by the downstream damming of the Cumberland River.

The trail becomes hard to follow at this point. Leave the river batteries and climb uphill on the road toward the log-hut replicas, which are modeled after those that housed

Confederate soldiers but were burned down after the Union took over to fight a measles outbreak. Turn left on the road that leads to the Luncheon Area, which is the first picnic area I've ever seen referred to in this way. Reach the picnic area and look for a huge oak tree backed by earthworks. The trail picks up again here, descending to a ravine along more earthworks (look for a hiker symbol on a small brown sign). The path is mowed as it passes through an open field. Heading south, soon reenter woods and climb to enter a thick pine grove. At mile 2.4, make a sharp left onto an old roadbed. Then pass through low woods before leaving right from the roadbed and climbing to another pine grove.

At mile 2.7, reach a trail junction. Here, Spur Trail leads left 1.3 miles to the Fort Donelson National Cemetery. Donelson Trail turns right in south-facing hickory–oak woods, then dives into a ravine. Cross an intermittent streambed on a footbridge, then climb out of the ravine by switchbacks. Shortly reach the backside of the visitor center and complete the loop.

Nearby Activities

Fort Donelson National Battlefield has an interesting museum and historical information. The Confederate Earthworks Walk, which is part of Fort Donelson, is also detailed in this book (see page 19). For more information, please visit **nps.gov/fodo**.

GPS TRAILHEAD COORDINATES

N36° 28.923' W87° 51.775'

From Exit 11 on I-24, northwest of downtown Nashville, take TN 76 for 3.4 miles west to a traffic light in Clarksville. TN 76 then becomes US 41A North. Continue on US 41A North 7.9 miles to US 79. Turn left on US 79 South and follow it 31.4 miles to reach Fort Donelson National Battlefield, just past the town of Dover, on your right. Park at the visitor center. Donelson Trail starts near the cannon to your left as you look outward from the visitor center.

23 Henry Hollow Loop

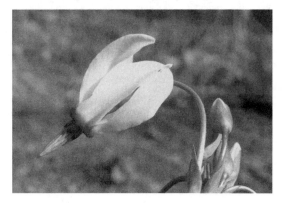

A shooting star is one of many spring wildflowers in Henry Hollow.

In Brief

This path is the gem of Beaman Park. It shows off the high and the low of this northwest Nashville preserve. Start along clear Henry Creek and ascend a deeply cut hollow full of wildflowers and other moisture-loving species. The path then heads to the oak-covered ridgetops before returning to the low end of Henry Hollow near Little Marrowbone Creek.

Description

Beaman Park is the setting for the Henry Hollow Trail, a first-rate spring wildflower destination. If you visited this park once a week starting in late March, you would see new wildflowers—including spring beauties, trillium, phlox, trout lily, toothwort, shooting stars, Jacob's ladder, dwarf crested iris, and more—blooming every trip. Summer and fall bring their share of flowers too. You can learn more at the informative nature center.

This path begins at the Creekside Trailhead of Beaman Park. While here, notice the shortleaf pines around the parking area; these trees are uncommon in Middle Tennessee. Leave the stone gateway trailhead on a gravel path bordered by more pines to reach a stone semicircle overlooking Henry Creek. The path turns up the creek and immediately reaches a trail junction and the loop portion of the Henry Hollow Trail. Continue along the creek, a crystalline stream spilling over layer upon layer of exposed shale that extends across the creek in thin panes. This unspoiled stream is typical of those that drain the Highland Rim surrounding the Nashville Basin. Stay above the creek, passing a contemplation bench. Beech, sycamore, dogwood, and redbud trees shade Henry Creek below, which flows in a wide sparkling sheet on sunny winter days. Intermittent wet-weather branches cut across the trail, diving for Henry Creek. After rains, the feeder branches, also with exposed layers

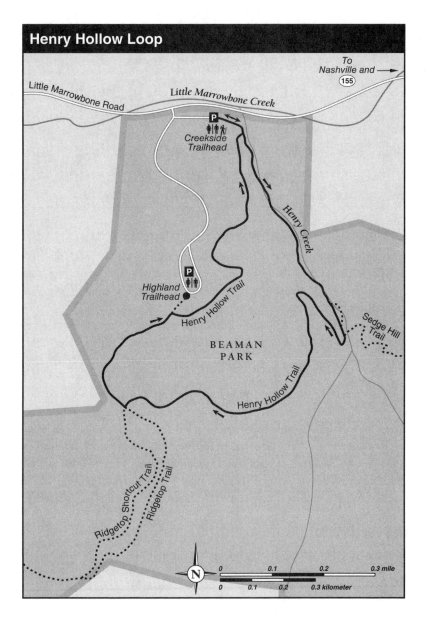

of shale, turn into noisy waterfalls. At 0.4 mile, the path spans such a feeder branch on a wooden bridge. Look across the creek for more feeder branches. The streams of Henry Hollow feed Little Marrowbone Creek, which runs along the road reaching the park. Little Marrowbone Creek then meets Marrowbone Creek near Ashland City before the pair of streams flows into the Cumberland River.

Ahead, the main trail continues forward, and a little spur path veers left along Henry Creek. Here, water and time have cut a big overhang in the rock across the creek, one

DISTANCE AND CONFIGURATION: 2.1-mile loop	**ACCESS:** No fees or permits required
DIFFICULTY: Moderate	**PETS:** On leash only
SCENERY: Streamside woods, ridgetop woods	**MAPS:** USGS *Forest Grove;* at trailside kiosk and at **tinyurl.com/beamanparknc**
EXPOSURE: Mostly shaded	**FACILITIES:** Restroom, picnic tables at parking area, nature center at park
TRAFFIC: Busy on weekends	**CONTACT:** 615-862-8580; **tinyurl.com/beamanparknc**
TRAIL SURFACE: Dirt and rocks	
HIKING TIME: 1.75 hours	**LOCATION:** Ashland City

reminiscent of rock formations on the Cumberland Plateau. A feeder branch cuts into Henry Creek just upstream of the overhang, creating low stairstep cascades on Henry Creek. The creek gathers in shallow pools where minnows dart away as you near them. Look in the water for crawdads, too, with their pincers ready to capture prey. Kids could have a blast playing in Henry Creek.

At 0.5 mile, Sedge Hill Trail leaves left 0.6 mile for the Beaman Park Nature Center, while Henry Creek Trail leaves Henry Creek and turns up the hillside to your right, using a pair of switchbacks to ease the grade. Watch for more wildflowers as the trail works up this steep slope to make a four-way trail junction at 1.3 miles. You are now in oak woods. Here, Ridgetop Trail goes to the left, and Ridgetop Shortcut Trail continues forward. To the right, Henry Hollow and Highland Trails run in conjunction with one another to reach a second junction at 1.5 miles; you'll see the Highland Trailhead at this second junction.

Henry Hollow Trail curves off the ridgetop, working along an oak-dominated, south-facing slope. The open woods are completely different here compared with the lush creek-side forest. The trail continues easing into Henry Hollow, eventually returning to bottomland and reaching a trail junction at 2 miles. From here, retrace your steps back to the trailhead.

Nearby Activities

Guided hikes and other programs are held periodically at Beaman Park. Check the park nature center or **tinyurl.com/beamanparknc** for more information. Ridgetop Trail is also located at Beaman Park (see page 113).

GPS TRAILHEAD COORDINATES
N36° 16.375' W86° 54.283'

From Exit 204 on I-40, west of downtown Nashville, take TN 155 North/Briley Parkway to Exit 24 (Ashland City/TN 12). Head east on TN 12 South and follow it 0.4 mile to Eatons Creek Road. Turn left on Eatons Creek Road and follow it 5 miles to Little Marrowbone Road. Turn left on Little Marrowbone Road and follow it 0.6 mile to Beaman Park on your left. The Creekside Trailhead is immediately to the left once you enter the park.

24 Hidden Lake Double Loop

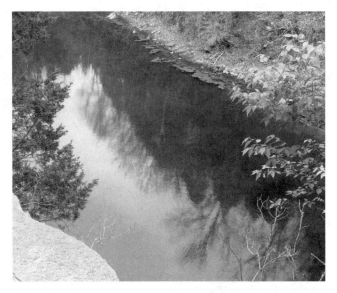

Even though you expect it, coming upon Hidden Lake is still a surprise.

In Brief

This hike takes place on one of nine separate tracts that comprise Harpeth River State Park. It travels through transitioning fields before entering woodland to reach bluffs above the Harpeth River. The trail then straddles the bluffs, with the Harpeth on one side and Hidden Lake on the other, before looping around a wooded knob past a tourist resort.

Description

Leave the open gravel parking area and enter a field to follow a grassy track toward Hidden Lake. A separate route heads downhill toward Harpeth River and is a canoe and kayak access point. Travel northwest through open terrain scattered with bird boxes. This former pasture is being managed for songbirds. The Harpeth River flows to your left beyond the screen of trees in the lower floodplain. At 0.2 mile, you'll reach a trail junction. Here, the Bluebird Loop heads right through the field. This will be your return route. For now, keep straight into the woodland, ambling on an old roadbed beside a small creek to your left. This up-and-coming forest is favorable for birds. It offers a mixture of young trees, bushes, and waterside habitat that all make for a rich ecosystem—the more habitat variety, the more species that can enjoy it. At 0.4 mile, the trail abruptly curves left and uses an old bridge to cross the creek along which you've been walking. Hackberry trees border the trail here.

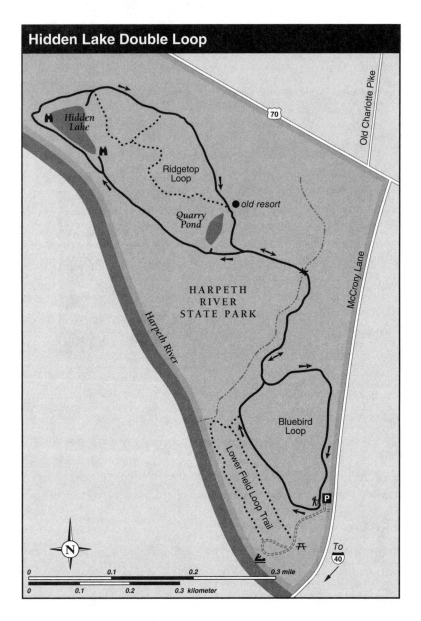

Hidden Lake Double Loop

You'll reach another trail intersection at 0.5 mile. Stay left, heading toward Hidden Lake. Just ahead, a spur trail leads right and uphill to a small quarry pond. Here you'll find contemplation benches and stone foundations from a forgotten building. Continue toward Hidden Lake. The old roadbed you are following is bordered by Harpeth River bottomland to your left and a steep hillside to your right. Also on your right, watch for a high bluff that is actually exposed stone from another quarry, albeit without a lake below it.

At 0.7 mile, you'll reach Hidden Lake. The roadbed heads to the silent waters surrounded by cut-rock walls. The trail cuts left and becomes a slender footpath ascending a

DISTANCE AND CONFIGURATION: 1.6-mile figure eight	**ACCESS:** No fees or permits
DIFFICULTY: Easy–moderate	**PETS:** On leash only
SCENERY: Rock bluffs, old quarry, cedar forest	**MAPS:** USGS *Kingston Springs;* at **tnstate parks.com/parks/about/harpeth-river**
EXPOSURE: Mostly shady	**FACILITIES:** None
TRAFFIC: Moderate on weekends	**CONTACT:** 615-952-2099; **tnstateparks**
TRAIL SURFACE: Grass, rocks, dirt, leaves	**.com/parks/about/harpeth-river**
HIKING TIME: 1 hour	**LOCATION:** Kingston Springs

rocky ridgeline dividing the Harpeth River from Hidden Lake, a large quarry pond. When you reach a rock prominence, you'll enjoy good views into Hidden Lake. You are literally walking a stacked rock spine that drops off in both directions. There is nothing else like it in this guide.

Finally, the trail slips over to the left side of the rock spine, ascends, and begins circling Hidden Lake, passing a vista looking south into the lake. Watch for cactus growing in the dry rocks. At 0.8 mile, you'll arrive at a four-way junction. To your far right, stone steps lead to the water's edge. To your right, a trail shortcuts the loop. Keep straight to make the longest loop possible and trace a roadbed to another junction at 0.9 mile. Again, continue heading straight to reach yet another junction at 1.1 miles. Check out the remains of an old 1940s resort; if you peer through the woods to your right, the quarry pond lies below. An examination of the building reveals no pioneer cabin but rather a "newer" old place. The structure itself is concrete block covered with finishing concrete on the outside. A water tank, electrical hookups, and more reveal the modernity of the structure. Look for the basketball rim around which an ancient cedar tree has grown. Shortly, you'll complete Ridgetop Loop and begin backtracking toward the trailhead. At 1.4 miles, you'll reach the Bluebird Loop. Turn left here, meandering through the field near McCrory Lane before completing the loop at 1.6 miles.

Nearby Activities

The Hidden Lake Tract of Harpeth River State Park also has a canoe launch, and the Harpeth River is ready and available for floating. You can also visit the Newsom Mill Tract of Harpeth River State Park. For more information, visit **tnstateparks.com/parks/about /harpeth-river**.

GPS TRAILHEAD COORDINATES
N36° 5.273' W87° 1.472'
From Exit 192 on I-40, take McCrory Lane north 0.9 mile, crossing the Harpeth River, and immediately look left for the trailhead parking area.

25 Johnsonville State Historic Park Loop

In Brief

Set along the banks of the Tennessee River, this hike loops through an area that was once a town, a railroad, and a Civil War battle site. Now dammed as Kentucky Lake, the hilly terrain along the lake provides an attractive setting for this walk into Tennessee history.

Description

Just a minor steamboat stop before the Civil War, the landing at Johnsonville was taken over by the Union and converted to a river-rail transfer point. During this time, the Union had also built a railroad connecting this landing to Nashville, enabling movement of supplies from the North by water and land. By train from Johnsonville, supplies were delivered to Nashville and south to Atlanta, where Sherman was preparing his ruthless March to the Sea.

Things looked grim for the rebels in November 1864. Their best chance was to cut off Union supplies and force the Union soldiers to retreat from Georgia to keep a safe supply line. Tennessee's General Nathan Bedford Forrest decided to attack and take Johnsonville to cut off the supply route and turn the South's sinking fortunes of war.

Forrest came north from Paris Landing on the Tennessee River, having captured a couple of Union boats; other cavalry members came by land. The general set up cannons at Pilot Knob, across the river from Johnsonville. On November 4, 1864, his small forces annihilated the Union's naval forces around Johnsonville, destroying 3 gunboats, 11 transports, 18 barges, and millions of dollars' worth of Union supplies.

This is the only time in recorded history that men on horses engaged and defeated a naval force. The engagement was a success for the South, but Sherman completed his March to the Sea, seizing supplies from citizens along the way. This march split the South in two and essentially ended the Civil War.

In 1945 the Tennessee Valley Authority bought the land for the damming of Kentucky Lake; Johnsonville was abandoned, and the railroad was rerouted.

Today, the area is a state park with hiking trails you can enjoy. The visitor center is also worth taking a look; it offers Civil War exhibits and a short film about the area's history. The visitor center is located on Nell Beard Road about 3 miles before you reach the main park entrance.

The trail system at Johnsonville State Historic Park adds up to 8 miles. At least that's what the park brochure states. You may have to make a few loops and double back to get all the miles in, but so what? Take your time looking around for clues of old homesites and signs of the town.

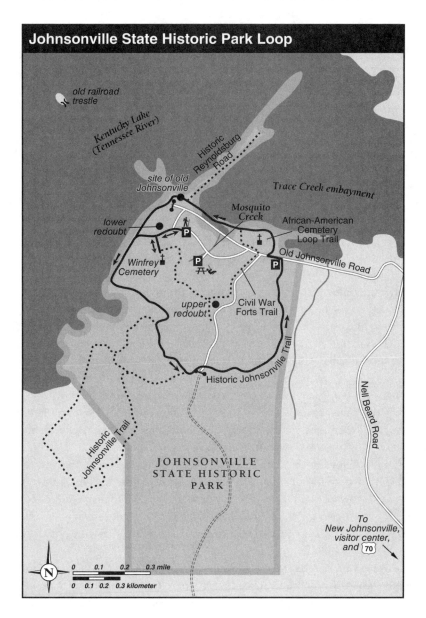

Johnsonville State Historic Park Loop

Start this loop northwest of the picnic area. Look for a narrow paved trail crossing a small culvert and ascending a hill into the woods. This path shortly crosses a paved road. Turn left to check out the Winfrey Cemetery. Oddly, the interment is situated inside the earthen defenses (redoubt) atop this hill. This redoubt was placed here to protect the rail and transfer point from the rebels.

As you are facing the trail sign, look to the right for a path entering young brush and woods; it is marked with a small wooden sign that reads TRAIL. These signs are placed

DISTANCE AND CONFIGURATION: 2.6-mile loop	**PETS:** On leash only
DIFFICULTY: Easy–moderate	**MAPS:** USGS *Johnsonville;* at **tnstate parks.com/parks/about/johnsonville**
SCENERY: Hardwood forest, huge lake	**FACILITIES:** Restrooms, water at picnic area
EXPOSURE: Mostly shady	
TRAFFIC: Not much	**CONTACT:** 931-535-2789; **tnstateparks .com/parks/about/johnsonville**
TRAIL SURFACE: Leaves, dirt, rocks, a little pavement	
HIKING TIME: 1.8 hours	**LOCATION:** New Johnsonville
ACCESS: No fees or permits	**COMMENTS:** This is one of many loop possibilities here.

along the path to keep you headed the right way. Follow this trail as it precipitously dives to an old roadbed paralleling the Tennessee River, now impounded as Kentucky Lake. Remember this point, as it will be part of your return route.

Turn left on the old roadbed and follow it along the river. The path shortly goes to the left from the roadbed and traverses a flat area of big hickories and oaks. Circle around the flat, crossing intermittent streambeds, to make a second trail junction at 0.7 mile. Turn left, heading up the hill that climbs steeply, and reach a contemplation bench where the trail levels off. Continue rambling through the woods to reach another trail junction at mile 1. Turn left here, and shortly reach the end of a paved turnaround.

Cross the paved road. The trail then dives into Meredith Hollow, where a clear stream makes a torturous course through the formerly settled flat. Daffodils abound in early March. Note that this area can be mucky.

Continue following the trail down Meredith Hollow to reach the park entrance road and alternate trailhead. Turn left, walk a short distance, and look for a trail entering the woods to your right. Continue in this marshy area and reach the raised railbed fought over by Forrest and the Union. Trace the railroad grade left, as you circle a little knob to your left. Leave the railbed near some stoneworks and emerge onto a dirt road, where you'll turn right.

The Trace Creek embayment is to your right. Pass the site of a railroad turntable on your left in the marsh of Mosquito Creek. Soon a paved road turns left up to the cemetery. Keep forward to reach the Johnsonville town site. Ahead, the raised railbed leads into the Tennessee River.

After looking around, continue on the roadbed past a metal gate. A steep hill, where the redoubt is, stands to your left. Kentucky Lake is to your right. The high point across the water, with a building atop it, is Pilot Knob. Continue and look for the trail leading left up to the redoubt (you came down this one). Climb the hill, pass the Winfrey Cemetery on your right, and pick up the narrow paved path down to your car.

GPS TRAILHEAD COORDINATES

N36° 3.694' W87° 57.903'

From Exit 172 on I-40, west of Nashville, take TN 46 North 4.4 miles to US 70 Business West near Dickson. Stay on US 70 Business West 1.3 miles to US 70 West. Turn left and stay on US 70 West 32.7 miles to Nell Beard Road. Turn right on Nell Beard Road and follow it 2.3 miles to Old Johnsonville Road. Turn left on Old Johnsonville Road and follow it 0.3 mile to the park entrance. Pick up a trail map at the entrance, continue 0.3 mile on the paved road, and park at the back of the lower picnic area. The hike starts on the narrow paved trail at the rear of the parking area.

26 Montgomery Bell Northeast Loop

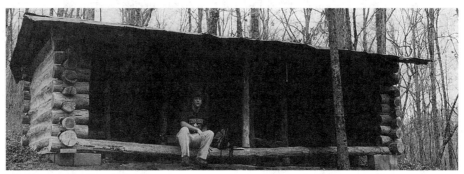

Wildcat Hollow trail shelter

In Brief

This loop traverses varied terrain, showing off the natural beauty Montgomery Bell State Park has to offer. It passes through rich hickory–oak woods, along clear streams, over ridges, and beside a lake. You can enjoy this hike in all seasons.

Description

Start the northeastern loop from the park office. Walk back toward the park entrance on the main park road, crossing Wildcat Creek on the road bridge. Shortly reach the old park headquarters building on your right. Pick up the MB Trail just beyond the building. Scramble up the hillside, and then pick up an old woods road. Begin a moderate but steady ascent through an oak–hickory forest on a narrow singletrack path. An observant eye will notice the older trees that bordered the old road. These contrast with the relatively younger trees growing on the old roadbed.

Pass near a pair of steep, deep hollows on your right before making a hard right at mile 1. Begin working your way down toward Wildcat Hollow, passing a small feeder branch, then reaching Wildcat Creek. Descend along Wildcat Creek and arrive at a large feeder stream at mile 1.4. Step over this stream. Dead ahead, up the hill, is the Wildcat Hollow trail shelter, used by backpackers for overnight camping trips. It overlooks the confluence of Wildcat Creek and its unnamed feeder branch.

From the shelter, MB Trail heads upstream in the hollow of the large feeder branch, crossing it twice. The creek begins to break up into small feeder branches of its own as it ascends the lush hollow. At mile 2.1, MB Trail turns away from the hollow and ascends a ridge as it stays inside park boundaries. The concrete park-boundary markers you see have been there since the park's inception in the 1930s.

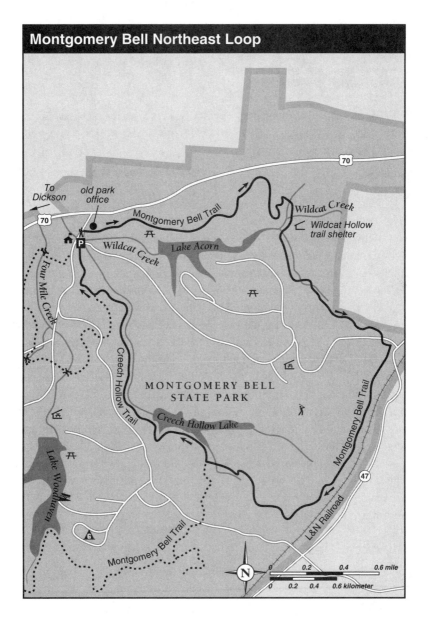

Montgomery Bell Northeast Loop

At mile 2.5, you'll come to a gravel park-service road. Turn left and follow the road toward TN 47, just beyond the gate you see ahead. The MB Trail turns right before reaching the gate and reenters woodland on a newer road that's sometimes used by park personnel to maintain the park's golf course, off to the right.

The walking is easy among the pines and cedars that grow alongside the ubiquitous oaks. Side trails leave to the right, toward the golf course. At mile 3.5, the MB Trail abruptly leaves the roadbed and turns right into a hollow; this turn is signed and hard to miss. Descend along this hollow, which, with the help of a few other small streams,

DISTANCE AND CONFIGURATION: 6-mile loop	**PETS:** On leash only
DIFFICULTY: Moderate	**MAPS:** USGS *Burns;* at park office and at **tnstateparks.com/parks/about /montgomery-bell**
SCENERY: Hardwood forest, creeks, lake	
EXPOSURE: Mostly shady	**FACILITIES:** Water, picnic tables, restroom at park office
TRAFFIC: Some on weekends	
TRAIL SURFACE: Leaves, dirt, rocks	**CONTACT:** 615-797-9052; **tnstateparks .com/parks/about/montgomery-bell**
HIKING TIME: 3 hours	
ACCESS: No fees or permits required	**LOCATION:** Burns

eventually gathers enough water to feed Creech Hollow Lake. The MB Trail stays along the edge of the hollow before descending to cross the stream that flows through the hollow. Climb away from the stream to reach a trail junction at mile 4.1. Then turn right, as the outer loop of the MB Trail goes to the left and circles the entire park. This other section of the MB Trail is part of the Montgomery Bell Southwest Loop (see page 103).

The cutoff MB Trail now runs with the orange-blazed Creech Hollow Trail. Descend to the shores of Creech Hollow Lake and skirt the lake's edge in woods to reach a clearing near the dam. Walk along the lake through the clearing and enter forest on the left side of the lake dam. Drop into the heart of Creech Hollow far below the lake level. A steep bluff flanks the trail, enabling you to grab views of the stream below.

Turn away from Creech Hollow, climbing a ridge to make a trail junction at mile 5.4. Then turn right at the junction, leaving the Creech Hollow Trail behind. Continue along the hardwood ridgeline before reaching a part of the park that looks like it was dug out at one time—it was. Take the wooden steps into an old rock quarry, now covered in pine trees. The stonework you see around the park came from this quarry. Continue beyond the quarry, and you'll soon reach a trail junction. Look across the park road for the park office, returning to the trailhead and completing the loop after 6 miles.

Nearby Activities

Montgomery Bell has a campground, mountain biking trails, fishing lakes, picnic areas, an inn, a restaurant, and a golf course. For more information, visit **tnstateparks.com /parks/about/montgomery-bell.**

GPS TRAILHEAD COORDINATES

N36° 6.073' W87° 16.985'

From Exit 182 on I-40, west of Nashville, head west on TN 96 for 10.5 miles to US 70 near Dickson. Turn right on US 70, and head 3.7 miles east to the state park entrance, which will be on the right. Enter and park at the office on your right. The loop begins on the main park road near the old park headquarters.

27 Montgomery Bell Southwest Loop

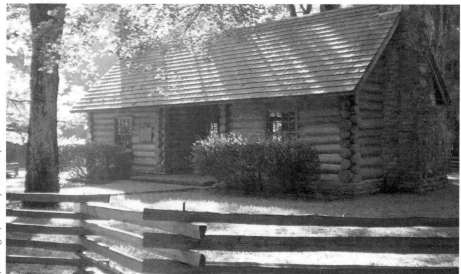

A replica of the Sam McAdow Cabin

In Brief

This hike explores southwestern Montgomery Bell State Park, making a long loop. First, tread among old pits from an 1800s iron-ore mine. Then pass a historic cabin site where a church denomination was founded and a local cemetery is still in use. Next, you'll see the natural beauty at Hall Spring, Lake Woodhaven, and Creech Hollow Lake.

Description

This loop hike is an exemplary woodland walk. The terrain is never difficult, and plenty of places beckon hikers to stop, linger, and contemplate nature and history. Pack a lunch and make a full day of it. Start the hike on the Montgomery Bell (MB) Trail, which leaves the Church Hollow Picnic Area and crosses the road on which you came. The MB Trail is blazed in white, and the Ore Pit Trail is blazed in red. These trails run together for the first and very last portion of the hike.

Head up a hill into a forest of oak, maple, and tulip trees on an old wagon road. You'll reach a trail junction at 0.2 mile and will immediately notice many holes in the ground. These holes, now rounded with time and grown over with trees, are the remains of pits

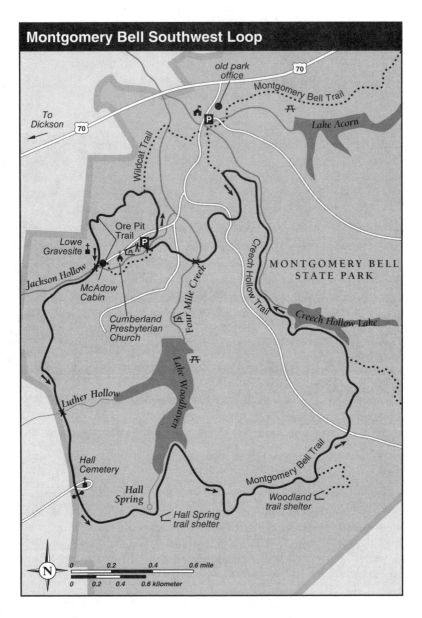

Montgomery Bell Southwest Loop

that were dug to extract the area's iron ore, which was fed into Laurel Furnace, located near the picnic area. Trees were cut and turned into charcoal to heat the ore, and water power was used to run a large bellows that blew oxygen into the fire. The molten iron was poured into molds known as sows, giving rise to the name pig iron. The discarded left-over material was slag. Most of these furnaces operated 24 hours a day, seven days a week. Can you imagine the heat of these furnaces in summer?

The MB Trail turns left at the junction. This path and park were named for Tennessee's premier iron industrialist of the early 1800s, Montgomery Bell. He established furnaces all

DISTANCE AND CONFIGURATION: 6.9-mile loop	**PETS:** On leash only
DIFFICULTY: Moderate	**MAPS:** USGS *Burns;* at park office and at **tnstateparks.com/parks/about /montgomery-bell**
SCENERY: Woods, creeks, lakes	
EXPOSURE: Nearly all shady	**FACILITIES:** Water at picnic area; picnic tables, restroom at park office
TRAFFIC: Moderate	
TRAIL SURFACE: Dirt, rocks, leaves	**CONTACT:** 615-797-9052; **tnstateparks .com/parks/about/montgomery-bell**
HIKING TIME: 4 hours	
ACCESS: No fees or permits required	**LOCATION:** Burns

over the area. Look around as the path winds between these old pits. The woods, dotted with tall white oaks, display the enduring healing powers of nature. Head downhill and reach a trail junction at mile 1. Here, a side trail leads 75 yards up an old wagon road to the lone grave of Dorothy Lowe, daughter of Sam and Jo Lowe. The girl lived just two years in the early 1900s. After the iron furnaces went cold, the Lowe family most likely farmed this area.

The MB Trail continues downhill and soon reaches a clearing and a cabin. This cabin is a replica of the one in which Sam McAdow, a founder of the Cumberland Presbyterian Church, lived. Back in 1810, a Christian revival swept rural areas of the country, and doctrinal differences led McAdow and others to form their own denomination. This cabin has two rooms separated by a dogtrot, which helped keep the cabin cooler in summer by allowing plenty of shade and dividing the kitchen, with its constant cooking fires, from the bedroom. Notice the giant sugar maples circling the cabin. Just down the field is a chapel that holds services on summer weekends.

The MB Trail passes beyond the cabin and over a clear stream on a footbridge. Look to the left just beyond the bridge at McAdow Spring. The squared-off stones still remain from days when the McAdows drew water from this source. Keep upstream on the creek that forms Jackson Hollow. Soon pass a concrete marker placed here by the National Park Service, which used this park as a recreation-demonstration project before it was handed over to the state of Tennessee. The MB Trail narrows and rises above the creek and swings around a fern-cloaked hill before leaving Jackson Hollow up a wagon road on a side branch.

Top out on a hill at mile 1.8, and find a resting bench. Descend along the park border to lushly vegetated Luther Hollow, crossing a clear stream on a footbridge with handrails. Climb sharply from Luther Hollow and level out to reach a gravel road at mile 2.5. To your left are a cedar-studded field and the Hall Cemetery, which is still used by local residents. Cross the gravel road, passing around a metal gate, to pick up an old woods road flanked by cedar and dogwood. Drop into a hardwood flat, crossing an often dry streambed on a footbridge, before reaching the Hall Spring trail shelter; backpackers use this site. Hall Spring is below the shelter and sends forth an estimated 1,000 gallons of water per minute from a large circular pool. The coolness and clarity of the water are indisputable.

Climb away from the trail shelter and turn north, following translucent Hall Creek past a closed wetland walkway, to reach the shores of the clear Lake Woodhaven, one of three impoundments that dot the state park. Follow the Hall Creek arm of the lake to a vista point and enjoy the view before turning away from the stream along a branch feeding the lake. Eventually, step over this branch and traverse a piney ridgeline. Drop into another drainage and small stream crossing, and then make a trail junction at mile 4.2. Here, a side trail leads right for a 10-minute walk to the Woodland trail shelter, another backpacker's campsite set on a hill above a rock-enclosed spring. Occasional yellow signs note that the land adjacent to the trail is being preserved as a Tennessee Natural Area.

The MB Trail climbs through hickory–oak woods to reach a park road at mile 4.5. At the trail junction at mile 4.8, turn left, as the outer loop of the MB Trail turns right and circles the entire park. The cutoff MB Trail now runs with the orange-blazed Creech Hollow Trail. Descend to reach the shores of Creech Hollow Lake, and skirt the lake's edge to reach a clearing near the dam. Continue along the lake through the clearing and enter the woods on the left side of the lake dam. Then drop into the heart of Creech Hollow far below lake level. A steep bluff flanks the trail.

Turn away from Creech Hollow, climbing a ridge, to make a trail junction at mile 6.1. Turn left here, leaving the Creech Hollow Trail behind. The MB Trail, which runs along the ridge before crossing a park road, undulates steeply across two dry ravines before making the most precipitous descent of the hike to reach Four Mile Creek. Span the creek on a footbridge, and then head downstream. Note the bluffs across the glassy watercourse. Turn away from the creek, passing a maintenance area and backpacker parking area. Climb into maple–cedar woods before crossing a paved road leading to Lake Woodhaven. You'll enter a full-blown cedar forest before intersecting the Ore Pit Trail again at mile 6.8. Turn right and descend, bridging a small stream, to enter the Church Hollow Picnic Area and complete the loop.

Nearby Activities

Montgomery Bell has recreation beyond its trail system. It offers a good campground, mountain biking trails, fishing lakes, picnic areas, an inn, a restaurant, and a golf course. You could incorporate any of the above with a hike.

GPS TRAILHEAD COORDINATES
N36° 5.058' W87° 17.268'

From Exit 182 on I-40, west of Nashville, head west on TN 96 for 10.5 miles to US 70 near Dickson. Turn right on US 70, and head 3.7 miles east to the state park entrance, which will be on the right. Enter the park and drive 0.5 mile to a fork in the road by a ball field. Take the right fork, drive just a short distance, and then take the next right toward Church Hollow. Park in the picnic area, which will be on your left.

28 Narrows of Harpeth Hike

In Brief

This hike travels along the Harpeth River, passing through an area known as the Narrows. Here, the Harpeth River, in a 5-mile-long bend, nearly curves back on itself. Highlights include a man-made tunnel that cuts across the bend in the river and panoramic views of the Harpeth River and the surrounding countryside.

Description

This is one of the more popular units of Harpeth River State Park. Here, visitors can float the Harpeth River, picnic and fish on its banks, and hike its trails. Back in the early 1800s, as Montgomery Bell developed the iron-ore industry in Middle Tennessee, he searched for a place to build a water-powered mill on the banks of the Harpeth River. Bell noticed the location where the river made such a bend that it nearly doubled back on itself, separated only by a slender but steep bluff. What took one person in a boat 5 miles by water took another on foot a half hour to clamber over. In those 5 miles, the Harpeth dropped several feet. It was here that Bell saw the chance to harness waterpower for his iron-ore industry by diverting water from the river through a tunnel—if he could cut through that bluff.

Using slave labor, Bell undertook the project in 1819, boring a tunnel through the limestone bluff that is 8 feet high, 16 feet wide, and 290 feet long. Just think of the skill and fortitude needed to complete such a project using the tools available then. The ironworks around the Narrows are long gone, but water still flows through the tunnel.

Start this hike by looking for a sign that reads TRAIL TO NARROWS AT BRIDGE. Head down and past some boulders to a picnic area on the riverbank. The gravel bar below is the takeout point for paddlers enjoying the 5-mile trip around the Narrows. Turn

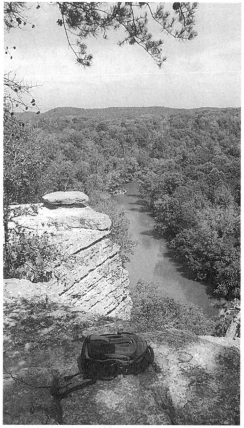

Grab a view from bluffs above the Harpeth River

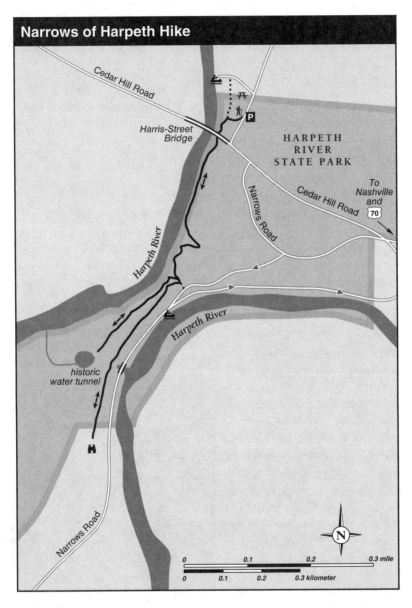

Narrows of Harpeth Hike

Cedar Hill Road

Harris-Street
Bridge

HARPETH
RIVER
STATE PARK

Cedar Hill Road

To
Nashville
and
70

Narrows Road

Harpeth River

Harpeth River

historic
water tunnel

Narrows Road

N

| 0 | 0.1 | 0.2 | 0.3 mile |
| 0 | 0.1 | 0.2 | 0.3 kilometer |

left, heading upstream on the Harpeth, and cross an intermittent streambed on a wooden bridge with handrails. The trail then heads under the Harris-Street Bridge and keeps upstream along the Harpeth, a good 50 feet above the river in cedar, oak, and maple woods; beard cane crowds the understory. Look out on the river where turtles may be lazing in the sun on logs. Soon you'll come to a rocky ravine; uphill to the left is a small rock house, and downhill the river is lined with small outcrops.

Continue and circle around a wooded ravine, crossing its low point on a bridge of cedar trunks. Ascend to walk along the base of a bluffline with many small rock houses.

DISTANCE AND CONFIGURATION: 1.8-mile out-and-back	**PETS:** On 6-foot leash only
DIFFICULTY: Easy	**MAPS:** USGS *Lillamay*; at **tnstateparks** **.com/parks/about/harpeth-river**
SCENERY: River, rock bluff, forest	**FACILITIES:** Picnic tables
EXPOSURE: Mostly shady	**CONTACT:** 615-952-2099; **tnstateparks** **.com/parks/about/harpeth-river**
TRAFFIC: Busy on weekends	
TRAIL SURFACE: Dirt, rocks	**LOCATION:** Kingston Springs
HIKING TIME: 1.3 hours	**COMMENTS:** This trail forks and has two out-and-backs; the 1.8 miles include both out-and-backs.
ACCESS: No fees or permits required	

Shortly, you'll reach a gap and trail junction at 0.4 mile. To your left, one trail leads a short distance to the canoe put-in. Another trail heads to the Narrows overlook. And a third trail leads right, downhill on an old wagon road toward the tunnel. Turn right and descend on the old wagon road into a flat where huge Eastern cottonwoods and sycamores tower over lush underbrush. Soon you'll reach the pool created by the outflow from Montgomery Bell's tunnel; this is a popular fishing hole. You can peer into the tunnel and appreciate the hard work that was required to make it.

Backtrack 0.2 mile to the previous trail junction and take the trail uphill to the overlook. Several wooden steps take you to the top of the bluff; then the walking is easy. Short side trails lead to the bluffline. Continue as the trail rises among shortleaf pine and cedar to a clear overlook 0.3 mile from the junction. Here, you can look down on the Harpeth River and the farm and hill country through which it flows. You can also see both sides of the Harpeth and, to the northeast, the white Harris-Street Bridge where you came from. On warm weekends, paddlers below drift down the river. The trail continues just a short distance beyond the overlook to dead-end at private property. Backtrack 0.6 mile to the trailhead.

Nearby Activities

Here at the Narrows of Harpeth, you can make a 5-mile canoe trip without needing a shuttle, using the trail described above. If you don't have a canoe, there are several liveries in the area, such as Tip-A-Canoe, **tip-a-canoe.com.**

GPS TRAILHEAD COORDINATES

N36° 9.147' W87° 7.099'

From Exit 188 on I-40, west of Nashville, take TN 249 North and follow it 2.3 miles to a T intersection with US 70. Turn left, heading west on US 70 for 2.3 miles to Cedar Hill Road. Turn right on Cedar Hill Road and follow it 3 miles to the Harris-Street Bridge, which will be on your right. Turn right just before the bridge to a parking area. The trail starts down by the Harpeth River beyond some vehicle-barrier boulders.

29 Nathan Bedford Forrest Five-Mile Trail

In Brief

This loop hike at Nathan Bedford Forrest State Park is an underused path at an underused state park. The terrain here will surprise you. Set among steep hills and deep hollows beside the wide Tennessee River, this trail is rich not only in natural beauty but in Tennessee history as well.

Description

Come to Nathan Bedford Forrest State Park if you're ready to embark on an adventurous mission from Nashville and learn a lot about the beauty and history of Tennessee. You have my guarantee as a native Tennessean that this 3,000-acre scenic swath will not disappoint. For starters, it has 20 miles of well-marked, well-maintained, little-trod trails. Hardwood-covered hills rise 300 feet above the Tennessee River. Clear streams cut through surprisingly steep hollows.

Pilot Knob is the beginning point for the trail system. This high point is named for its use as a point of reference for riverboat pilots plying the Tennessee River below. I will admit that this place is a little outside the 60-mile parameter of this book, but the trail system is too good to be overlooked.

Now, to the trails. A few of the shorter trails are isolated walks, and the rest are laid out in a series of interconnected loops. Loop hikes can range from 0.25 to 20 miles in length; backpackers use some of the longer loops for overnight camping. The following trail description is of the Five-Mile Trail. Adventurous hikers, however, can look at the park map and come up with loops of varying lengths. During winter and early spring, hikers will be able to enjoy river views. In spring, visitors will see wildflowers in the hollows. In the summer, hikers will want to hit the trail early in the morning.

Begin the Five-Mile Trail, marked with orange metal blazes, atop Pilot Knob. Descend northeast atop a steep and surprisingly narrow ridgeline shaded by tall oaks. Notice that the trail bed is often lined with moss. Winter views of the river are off to your right. Drift downward, finally curving into Chester Hollow, originally called Cherry Hollow. This area was named for a fellow named Cherry, who lent his name to all sorts of area landmarks. Later, some errant map maker named it Chester Hollow—and the name stuck.

The path heads up the southern side of Chester Hollow, crossing over streambeds draining Pilot Knob Ridge. Beech and tulip trees, along with omnipresent oaks, adorn the flat. Work up the hollow to make a trail junction at mile 1.5; signs indicate that the Five-Mile Trail keeps to the right. Stay right and head east, out of Chester Hollow, where fingerlike flats extend into the hills. You'll arrive near the Tennessee River, only to turn away. Hikers could cut through some trees to reach the water's edge. The trail then curves into

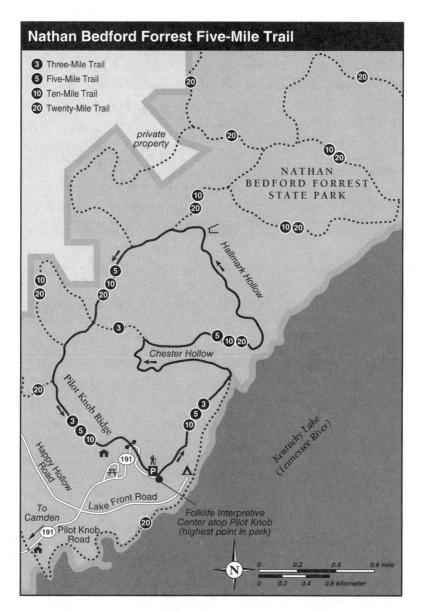

Hallmark Hollow, away from the river. Step over a few streambeds while working up the ever-narrowing hollow. Suddenly, the trail ascends a rib ridge to gain 200 feet in 0.1 mile. The rib ridge levels out to reach a backpacker's trail shelter at mile 2.8. Beyond this three-sided wooden structure, continue uphill at a more reasonable grade to soon arrive at a trail junction.

At the junction, the Five-Mile Trail turns left. Begin following the main ridgeline of the park, which roughly parallels the north–south direction of the Tennessee River that you can see in winter from this ridge. The path undulates to reach another junction at

DISTANCE AND CONFIGURATION: 4.9-mile loop	**PETS:** On leash only
DIFFICULTY: Moderate	**MAPS:** USGS *Johnsonville;* at visitor center and at **tnstateparks.com/parks**
SCENERY: Oak forests, shady hollows, big river	**/about/nathan-bedford-forrest**
EXPOSURE: Mostly shady	**FACILITIES:** Restrooms, water at visitor center
TRAFFIC: Not much, some on nice weekends	**CONTACT:** 731-584-6356; **tnstateparks** **.com/parks/about/nathan-bedford-forrest**
TRAIL SURFACE: Leaves, moss, rocks, dirt	**LOCATION:** Eva
HIKING TIME: 2.7 hours	**COMMENTS:** This is just one loop among 20-plus miles of trails here.
ACCESS: No fees or permits required	

mile 3.7. The Three-Mile Trail joins here, also returning to Pilot Knob. Follow the orange blazes forward. The ridgetop trail begins curving southeast onto Pilot Knob Ridge, and other roads join the main path. Parts of the wide, roadlike trail have been cleared. Pass a park resident cabin on your right at mile 4.4, and descend from the cabin area to reach Pilot Knob Road. Pass around the metal gate, cross the road, and begin climbing toward Pilot Knob. Soon join Pilot Knob Road for the last ascent to the parking area and the end of the Five-Mile Trail.

Nearby Activities

Nathan Bedford Forrest State Park makes for a great overnight destination, offering camping, cabins, and outdoor activities. Anglers and boaters love the proximity of Kentucky Lake. The Folklife Interpretive Center, atop Pilot Knob, provides interesting information about the riverboat days on the Tennessee and the life of Confederate General Nathan Bedford Forrest, who fought one of the Civil War's most fascinating battles in this vicinity. Furthermore, this state park has two excellent campgrounds, including one situated directly on the banks of the Tennessee River. Having written numerous campground guidebooks, I can say with authority that these sites are some of the finest in the Southeast.

GPS TRAILHEAD COORDINATES

N36° 5.323' W87° 58.455'

From Exit 172 on I-40, west of Nashville, take TN 46 North 4.4 miles to US 70 Business West near Dickson. Stay on US 70 Business West 1.3 miles to US 70 West. Turn left and stay on US 70 West 39.9 miles to US 70 Business West into the town of Camden. In 2.7 miles, from the town square at the Benton County Courthouse, take TN 191 North 7.8 miles to Nathan Bedford Forrest State Park. Stop at the park office and get a trail map. Continue beyond the park office 1 mile to the Interpretive Center atop Pilot Knob. The trail starts on the left side of the building.

30 Ridgetop Trail at Beaman Park

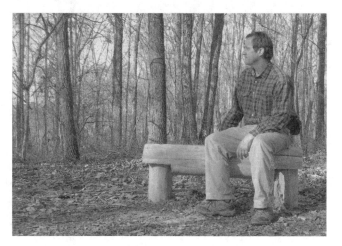

Author relaxes at a bench along the Ridgetop Trail.

In Brief

This ridge-running trail at Beaman Park winds through Highland Rim woodlands to end among big oaks. Never too steep, the path nevertheless offers views into incredibly precipitous hollows that cut deep into the Highland Rim.

Description

Ridgetop Trail at Beaman Park was a long time in the making. The 1,500-acre tract was purchased by the city of Nashville in 1996, and it took nearly 10 years from the time of purchase until the park was open for unsupervised visitation as it is today. Now a nature center has been added. Ridgetop Trail will show you that this part of Davidson County is rugged, steep, and still a little wild. It will also show you that Alvin Beaman, a former member of the city park board, would be proud of his wife's donation of the money to buy this slice of the Highland Rim. You will appreciate the group of doctors who sold the tract to the state at half its appraised value. This land, known to early Nashvillians as Paradise Ridge, for brothers named Paradise, is now a natural paradise where clear streams have cut surprisingly steep hollows divided by narrow ridges of hickory and oak, places where deer and turkey roam.

The park has been tastefully developed, as you will see at the trailhead where a stone entryway and kiosk serve as your corridor to the hike. Ridgetop Trail, true to its name, stays on the top of the ridgeline, meandering amid oaks aplenty. Descend from the trailhead to join

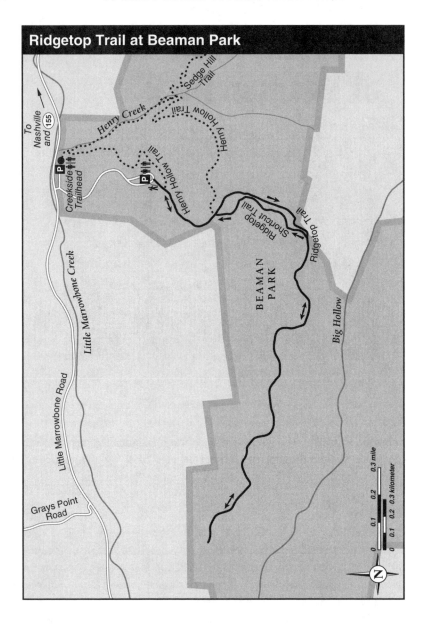

an old roadbed, and meet one end of Henry Hollow Trail. Stay with the red-blazed Ridge-top Trail as it drifts over to the south side of the ridge, skirting a deep hollow to your left.

The wide track soon reaches another trail junction: To your left, Henry Hollow Trail leads to Henry Creek; Ridgetop Trail Shortcut goes off to the right. Use the shortcut on your return. Continue on Ridgetop Trail. The dirt-and-rock track runs south amid young forest. At 0.6 mile, you'll reach old Blueberry Hill Road, a service road that goes off to the left. Blueberry Hill is yet another name this area had when it was a private hunting

DISTANCE AND CONFIGURATION: 4.2-mile out-and-back	**ACCESS:** No fees or permits required
	PETS: On leash only
DIFFICULTY: Moderate	**MAPS:** USGS *Forest Grove*; at trailside kiosk and at **tinyurl.com/beamanparknc**
SCENERY: Ridgetop woodlands	
EXPOSURE: Mostly shady	**FACILITIES:** Restroom, picnic tables at parking area; nature center at park
TRAFFIC: Moderate to busy on weekends	
	CONTACT: 615-862-8580; **tinyurl.com /beamanparknc**
TRAIL SURFACE: Dirt	
HIKING TIME: 2 hours	**LOCATION:** Ashland City

preserve. Ridgetop Trail keeps right. The young trees here reveal another use this land had—timber extraction. You are now on an old logging road.

In spring look for bluets and pussy toes, wildflowers that can grow in drier places such as this hickory–oak forest. Reach the other end of the Ridgetop Shortcut Trail in a gap at 0.8 mile. Look around here, and notice that on either side of you the land drops off precipitously. The trail climbs away from the gap in an area of many tulip trees. These trees often are the first to regenerate after an area has been cleared, as this ridge undoubtedly once was. In winter, you'll have views of the adjacent ridges divided by chasmlike streamsheds.

Ridgetop Trail continues a pattern of undulating between narrow gaps and knobs, heading west into more mature woods. At 2.1 miles, the trail ends at a level knob. Contemplation benches allow hikers to rest and relax while enjoying this reward. They can also contemplate hiking back 2.1 miles to the trailhead. On the return trip, try to see what you may have missed on the way in. Also, hikers should take Ridgetop Shortcut Trail while returning. The twisting, winding singletrack footpath actually isn't any shorter, but it covers new terrain and works around the edges of deep hollows. It also travels through moister woods, which offer more wildflowers in spring.

Nearby Activities

Guided hikes and other programs are held periodically at Beaman Park. Check the nature center or **tinyurl.com/beamanparknc** for more information. Henry Hollow Loop (see page 90) is also located at Beaman Park.

GPS TRAILHEAD COORDINATES

N36° 15.942' W86° 54.312'

From Exit 204 on I-40, west of downtown Nashville, take TN 155 North/Briley Parkway to Exit 24 (Ashland City/TN 12). Head east on TN 12 South and follow it 0.4 mile to Eatons Creek Road. Turn left on Eatons Creek Road and follow it 5 miles to Little Marrowbone Road. Turn left on Little Marrowbone Road and follow it 0.6 mile to Beaman Park on your left. The Ridgetop Trailhead is up the hill once you enter the park.

SOUTHWEST

INCLUDING COLUMBIA, FAIRVIEW, AND FRANKLIN

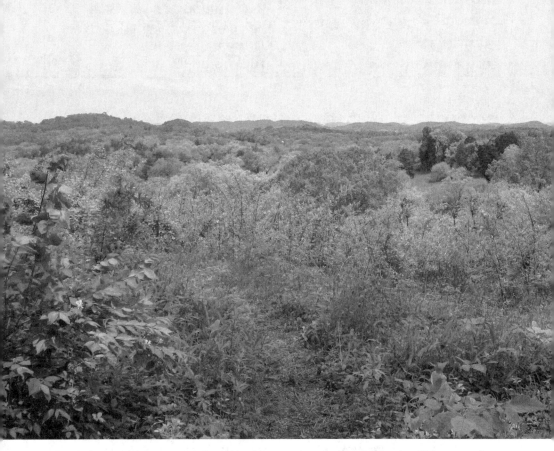

Confederate cannons were placed at this very view during the Battle of Thompson's Station (see page 125).

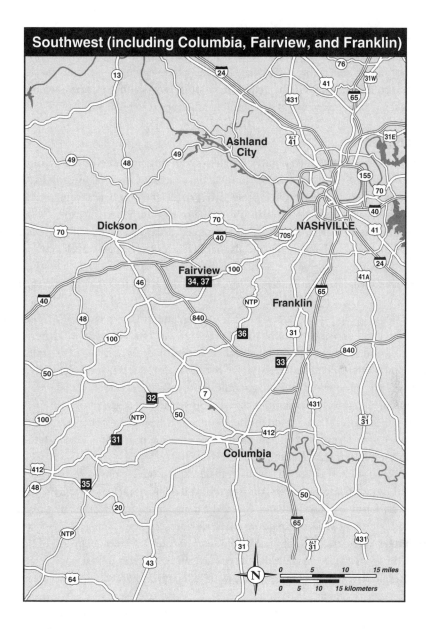

Southwest (including Columbia, Fairview, and Franklin)

31 Devil's Backbone Loop

In Brief

This hike traverses a lesser visited state natural area despite being conveniently located adjacent to the Natchez Trace Parkway. Making a loop through a seldom traveled hardwood forest, the path stays in the center of the preserve, exuding an aura of wildness that makes even wintertime views of surrounding hills appear to be the back of beyond.

Description

The name Devils Backbone conjures up an array of images—a hellish maze of rocks or maybe a menacing ridge of stone. But this name was actually inspired by the adjacent Natchez Trace. In the early 1800s, during the heyday of traveling the Trace from Natchez, Mississippi, to Nashville, an arduous trip was virtually assured. Flooded rivers, robbers, bad weather, hostile American Indians, and the rigors of day-after-day, self-propelled travel made the journey challenging. The perils that befell Natchez Trace travelers were said to be the work of the devil, and the Devils Backbone sprang up as a nickname for the Trace.

Today, Devils Backbone seems as little used as the original Trace was after the advent of steamboats. The site, protected as a Tennessee State Natural Area in 1997 and dedicated in 2001, has an excellent loop trail through upland forest types of the Western Highland Rim. The Tennessee Natural Areas Program was established in 1971 by the state legislature, and since then 62 state natural areas have been established. The state of Tennessee doesn't own all the lands; rather it works with local, state, and federal agencies, as well as private landowners, in managing these sites. The goal is to attain adequate representation of all natural communities that comprise the landscape of the Volunteer State and provide long-term protection for rare, endangered, and threatened plant and animal life. Little exotic-plant invasion and good representation of tree species make the Devils Backbone a superior state natural area.

A hiker-registration book is at the trailside kiosk. Make sure to register—the more visitors this state-owned area gets, the greater the likelihood that it will remain preserved. Enter a lush hardwood forest of mostly oaks on a singletrack path marked by white blazes. At 0.1 mile, the trail picks up an old woods road and turns left, slicing between steep and deep hollows. The trail bed of grass and moss indicates the infrequent use of this path, though the white blazes on trailside trees clearly mark the trail. It is easy to see why early Trace travelers stayed on the ridgelines, as trekking up and down the desiccated ravines would become tiresome.

At 0.4 mile, the loop portion of the trail begins. Stay right and work mostly downhill along another ridgeline. Notice that most of the trees here are chestnut oak, which is easily identified by its thick leaves with wavy edges. Chestnut oaks range from Maine to Mississippi, thriving in dry, rocky upland soils such as on this ridge. Since the demise of the

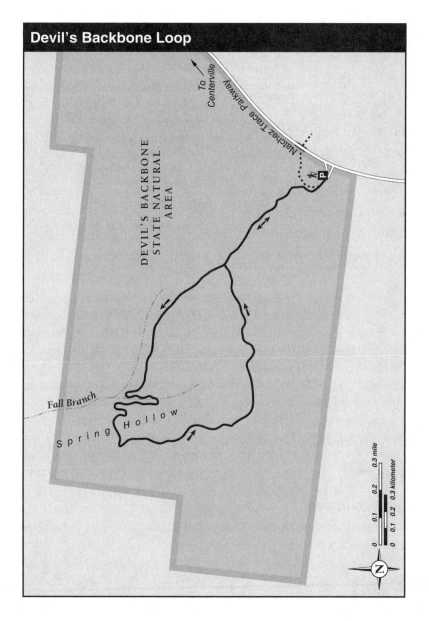

American chestnut, the chestnut oak's density and distribution has increased. Its nuts are favored by wildlife, and because of its high tannin content the bark was once used for tanning leather.

The trail descends into Spring Hollow, reaching Fall Branch. Circle back to the left and step over Fall Branch at mile 1. The clarity of the stream allows you to peer into the water and look for underwater life. Ahead, cross a feeder branch on a footbridge, and head up the hollow to step over a third branch. The trail then curves back down Spring

DISTANCE AND CONFIGURATION: 2.7-mile loop	**MAPS:** USGS *Gordonsburg;* at **tinyurl .com/devilsmap;** Natchez Trace Parkway map at **tinyurl.com/natcheznash**
DIFFICULTY: Easy–moderate	
SCENERY: Hardwood forest, creek-filled hollow	**FACILITIES:** Restrooms, water 15 miles north on Natchez Trace Parkway
EXPOSURE: Nearly all shady	**CONTACT:** Natchez Trace Parkway: 800-305-7417; **nps.gov/natr;** Devil's Backbone State Natural Area: 731-512-1369; **tn.gov/environment/article/na-na -devils-backbone**
TRAFFIC: You will likely have this trail to yourself.	
TRAIL SURFACE: Grass, moss, leaves, dirt	**LOCATION:** Hohenwald
HIKING TIME: 1.3 hours	
ACCESS: No fees or permits required	**COMMENTS:** Consider traveling 2.2 miles south on the Natchez Trace Parkway to enjoy Fall Hollow Trail too.
PETS: On 6-foot leash at all times	

Hollow—this path is one of exploration, not expediency. The bottomland is rife with wildflowers in spring. Beech trees, which shade the hollow, love well-drained, moist soils like those in Spring Hollow. In fall, squirrels, raccoons, and other mammals gorge on beechnuts. As is often seen, the smooth trunks of beech trees prove irresistible for some folks who like to carve dates and names in them.

Climb out of Spring Hollow by switchbacks, returning to the oak-dominated ridgeline at mile 1.4. Turn left onto an old roadbed. (The seemingly endless forest and distant hills radiate a wildness that belies the size of the 950-acre natural area.) Undulate along the ridgeline, looking down into the hollows where small streamlets gather and feed Big Swan Creek to the west. The path curves back to the east, intersecting the beginning of the loop at 2.3 miles. From here, turn right and backtrack 0.4 mile to the trailhead.

Nearby Activities

Just 2.1 miles south on the Natchez Trace is Fall Hollow Waterfall. A short paved trail leads to the top of this cascade.

GPS TRAILHEAD COORDINATES

N35° 36.333' W87° 24.375'

From Exit 192 on I-40, west of downtown Nashville, take McCrory Lane 4.4 miles south to intersect TN 100. Turn right and immediately pick up the Natchez Trace Parkway. Head south on the parkway 48.3 miles to the signed right turn into Devil's Backbone State Natural Area, on your right.

32 Gordon House and Ferry Site Walk

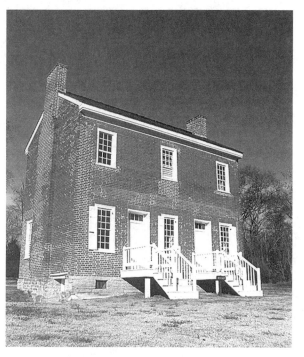

The Gordon House was built in 1817.

In Brief

This relatively short walk is laced with history. Located just off the Natchez Trace Parkway near Columbia on the banks of the Duck River, the trail first passes by the 200-year-old Gordon House. It then picks up a section of the Old Trace, following the actual route taken by Americans of long ago. The trail ends at the edge of the Duck River, where a ferry operated for nearly a century during the 1800s.

Description

The Natchez Trace follows an old path first used by buffalo and then by American Indians who followed the animals. Later, as the United States began to be settled, farmers floated their crops down the waterways of the greater Mississippi River Valley to Natchez,

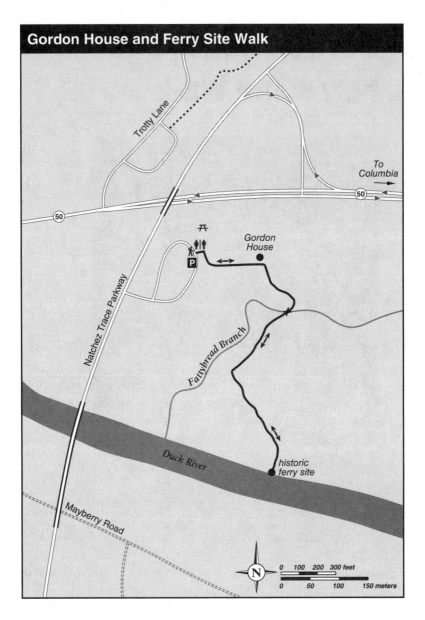

Gordon House and Ferry Site Walk

Mississippi, or New Orleans to be sold. The strong currents that brought their flatboats down the river prevented their return float home, and the boats were dismantled and sold for lumber. The farmers then had a long walk up this American Indian–buffalo path north to their homes.

The United States realized the economic importance of the path and improved it to encourage trade. In 1800 the U.S. Army began establishing an official "Natchez Trace," passing through American Indian lands in Mississippi, Alabama, and Tennessee. Along the way many inns, or stands as they were known, were established to feed and house travelers.

DISTANCE AND CONFIGURATION: 1-mile out-and-back	**PETS:** On 6-foot leash at all times
DIFFICULTY: Very easy	**MAPS:** USGS *Greenfield Bend;* at **nps.gov/natr/planyourvisit/upload**
SCENERY: Fields, hardwood forest, creek, river	**/Gordon-House-with-bleeds.pdf;** Natchez Trace Parkway map at
EXPOSURE: Mostly shady	**tinyurl.com/natcheznash**
TRAFFIC: Steady during good weather	**FACILITIES:** Restrooms, covered picnic tables at parking area
TRAIL SURFACE: Asphalt, dirt	
HIKING TIME: 30 minutes	**CONTACT:** 800-305-7417; **nps.gov/natr**
ACCESS: No fees or permits required	**LOCATION:** Williamsport

Around 1803, John Gordon, so-called Indian fighter and a friend of Andrew Jackson, obtained 600 acres along the Duck River in a land grant and began operating a ferry across the Duck near his homestead by the Old Trace. Before his ferry, travelers could cross the Duck only when it was low enough to be forded. In 1817, Gordon built himself and his wife a brick home, one of the first in the area. He died shortly after the home was built, but his wife continued to live there until her death in 1859. This is one of the few original buildings associated with the Old Trace.

Leave the parking area and follow the paved path to the Gordon House. The sturdy structure stands out on the landscape, no matter what the season, thanks in part to its white-paned windows that contrast with the red brick. John Gordon regularly saw the rise and fall of the Duck River through the seasons and smartly chose to build his home on this hill atop the floodplain.

The paved path ends at the house. Drop down the hill to your right, entering a grassy field where Gordon and his wife likely planted crops. Cross a bridge over Fattybread Branch. The origin of this watercourse's name has been lost to time. An attractive grassy flat lies on the far side of the stream, and a contemplation bench overlooks the creek as it makes a bend toward the Duck River.

Pick up the Old Trace on the far side of Fattybread Branch. You can be sure that the soldiers who built this part of the road in 1802 drank from the branch. Think of all the travelers who, either coming or going, had the crossing of the Duck River on their mind at this point. Follow the Old Trace as it passes over a hill and emerges onto another flat of grass broken by trees.

The trail skirts the edge of the flat and leads toward the Duck River. You'll reach a final level spot, which was the staging area for the ferry. Many a traveler, horseman, and farmer waited here. The dirt path continues down to the banks of the Duck. This usually clear, green, wide river is bordered with sycamore and hackberry.

Decades of off-and-on flooding have obliterated signs of the ferry operation, which ran from the early 1800s to 1896, when a bridge was built over the Duck. Gordon had to share his profits from the ferry with Chickasaw Chief George Colbert, who by treaty controlled ferries on American Indian lands. Now the Duck is easily crossed on the Natchez Trace Parkway and numerous other bridges. Life sure has changed over the past 200 years.

Nearby Activities

The Natchez Trace Parkway offers other hiking trails, historical information, camping, and more. The Natchez Trace National Scenic Trail is just north of the Gordon House on TN 50.

GPS TRAILHEAD COORDINATES

N35° 43.219' W87° 15.680'

From Exit 192 on I-40, west of downtown Nashville, take McCrory Lane 4.4 miles south to intersect TN 100. Turn right and immediately pick up the Natchez Trace Parkway. Head south on the parkway 34.4 miles to the Gordon House, on your left just past TN 50.

---

33 Heritage Park/Thompson's Station Park Hike

In Brief

This hike combines trails at two parks to make one good trek. Start at Heritage Park and wind your way up a wooded ridgeline; then descend to Thompson's Station Park, where you will follow a gravel track around a more traditional developed park. Climb back over the ridge and join a different path that leads past an overlook, once a Civil War cannon emplacement during the battle of Thompson's Station.

Description

Interestingly, not only does this hike connect two parks, but it also connects two major watersheds. The two parks, Heritage Park and Thompson's Station Park, are separated by a line of hills known as Duck River Ridge. To the south of the ridge, streams flow into the Duck River, part of the Tennessee River Basin, while streams north of Duck River Ridge flow north into the Harpeth River, a tributary of the Cumberland River Basin.

At the parks, Duck River Ridge rises 140 feet above the landscape, and the importance of being able to see out from here was not lost on Civil War soldiers. On March 5, 1863, Union forces were advancing from Franklin toward Thompson's Station. Confederate forces placed cannons atop this ridge facing north toward Thompson's Station. The Union was reconnoitering the area when they ran into rebels. The Confederates retreated, luring the Northerners in. The Union warily settled in for the night, but was bombarded by cannon fire from this very ridge during what seemed an interminable darkness. The next morning, the Yankees pushed forward, and a bloody hand-to-hand battle ensued. Part of the Union forces withdrew, and Confederate genius General Nathan Bedford Forrest saw an opening, then snuck around the remaining Yankees' north side, cutting off their escape. After more deadly battling, the federals eventually surrendered. Over a thousand men were taken prisoner. This slowed Union offensive forays into Middle Tennessee for a while.

Your exploration of Duck River Ridge is likely to be much less dangerous. The hike leaves north from the parking area at Heritage Park and follows concrete steps between ball field 4 and ball field 5. After cutting between the ball fields and passing a little concession stand, you will see a trail signboard and path entering woods. Enter a mix of hardwoods and cedars on a natural-surface path, Alexander Trail. At 0.1 mile, intersect Stephens Way, a winding track that switchbacks all along the south side of the ridge. That trail will be part of your return route, but for now stay straight with the Alexander Trail, heading uphill in youngish woods. Cross the tower/water tank access road at 0.3 mile. Look southeast for a surprisingly far-reaching view of the Duck River Valley. Enter a brushy area then full-blown woods. Cross Stephens Way a second time at 0.4 mile.

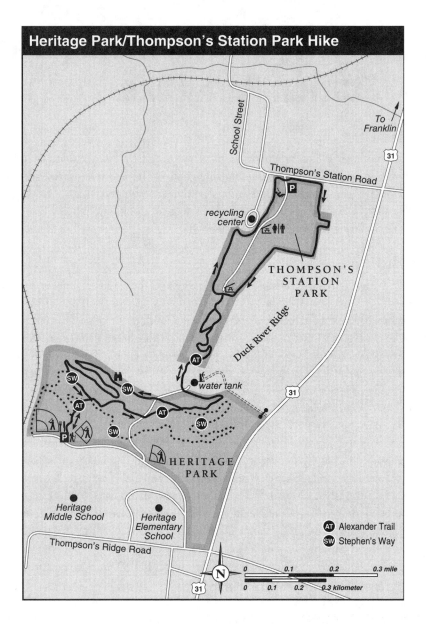

At 0.5 mile, make a hard switchback left, as a short trail leads right to a tower access road. Resume climbing and return to the tower access road at 0.6 mile. A pair of water tower tanks stands just to your right. The trail drops over the ridge in taller, more mature woods. Tulip trees and oaks grow big. Descend and stay left at a pair of miniloops before dropping to open grassy area and a picnic pavilion, now in Thompson's Station Park, at 0.9 mile. Head left here on a gravel track. Begin making a clockwise loop around

DISTANCE AND CONFIGURATION: 3-mile figure eight	**HIKING TIME:** 1.5 hours
DIFFICULTY: Moderate	**ACCESS:** No fees or permits required
SCENERY: Wooded ridge, park	**PETS:** On leash only
EXPOSURE: Mostly shady, some open sun	**MAPS:** USGS *Spring Hill;* at trailhead
TRAFFIC: Moderate, busier on gravel track at Thompson's Station Park	**FACILITIES:** Restrooms, picnic facilities at Thompson's Station Park
TRAIL SURFACE: Natural, gravel, a little pavement	**CONTACT:** outdoorencounter.org
	LOCATION: Thompson's Station

Thompson's Station Park. The trail becomes briefly paved at 1.1 miles, and you shortly come to the park entrance, where the path is back to gravel. There is alternate parking here, as well as a children's playground.

Walk very close to Thompson's Station Road before turning back south at 1.3 miles. The trail roughly parallels the park boundary. Return to the park pavilion at 1.7 miles. It is time to climb Duck River Ridge again, backtracking on Alexander Trail. Pass below the water tanks again at 2.1 miles, now officially on the south side of the hill. Finally return to new trail, joining Stephens Way at 2.3 miles. Keep west along the slope of the ridge. At 2.5 miles, a short spur leads right to the overlook and cannon emplacement site where the Confederates interrupted Yankee sleep the night before the Battle of Thompson's Station. Today, the view to the north is mostly of wooded hills beyond Thompson's Station. Continue west along the ridge, where Stephens Way makes long switchbacks downhill. At 2.8 miles, stay straight as a spur leads right heading to the west side of ball field 5. Before long you are back at Alexander Trail. Turn right and backtrack to the trailhead, completing the hike.

Nearby Activities

Heritage Park has ball fields and a concession area when the ball fields are open. Thompson's Station Park is more of a traditional park and has a picnic shelter, a playground, and other picnicking locations.

GPS TRAILHEAD COORDINATES

N35° 47.344' W86° 55.078'

From Exit 59 on I-65, south of Nashville, follow TN 840 West 2.9 miles. Take Exit 28, and head south on US 31 for 2.9 miles to a traffic light. Buckner Road goes left at the light, but you turn right at the light onto Thompsons Ridge Road. Go just a short distance on Thompsons Ridge Road to Heritage Elementary School; then immediately turn right again toward the ball fields. Continue almost to the end of the road to the steps leading down between ball field 4 and ball field 5.

34 Lakes of Bowie Loop

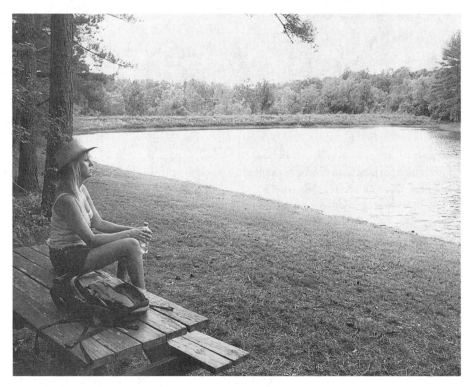

Overlooking Lake Anna on a cloudy summer day

In Brief

This loop hike encompasses several short scenic trails of Bowie Nature Park, touring four of the preserve's lakes. The trails have good footing, are mostly level and wide, and are suitable for a family hike, especially for younger children. Wildlife can be abundant as well, with waterfowl in the lakes, and deer and more in adjacent woods.

Description

This is a water- and wildlife-lover's walk that meanders by small lakes, beneath tall pines, and through quiet hollows. Take the Lake Van Trail, circling this attractive impoundment, and pick up the Loblolly Loop, passing by Upper Lake. Cross a spring branch to get to Lake Byrd and a picnic shelter. Circle by Lake Anna before returning to the trailhead, passing by Sycamore Springs, a chilly water source from the days when Bowie Nature Park was a farmstead.

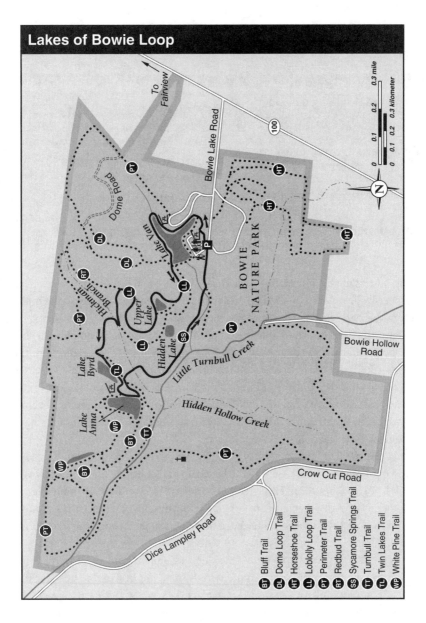

Lakes of Bowie Loop

Waterfowl enjoy the lakes, which also harbor fish and are open to fishing. Watch for land critters too. I have seen deer on nearly every visit here. Keep your eyes open as you walk along the shores of the lakes and edges where field and forest meet.

A number of trails wind through Bowie Nature Park; those in the heart of the park are designated as scenic trails. This hike traces a portion of the scenic trails, though you may want to create your own loop. In fact, there are so many small trails, you may make up your

DISTANCE AND CONFIGURATION: 2.2-mile loop	**ACCESS:** No fees or permits required; daily, sunrise–sunset
DIFFICULTY: Easy	**PETS:** Must be on a leash at all times
SCENERY: Small lakes, pine woods	**MAPS:** USGS *Craigfield*; at **bowiepark.org**
EXPOSURE: Part sun, part shade	**FACILITIES:** Water spigot, restrooms, picnic area at trailhead
TRAFFIC: Plenty of solitude during the week, some company on weekends	**CONTACT:** 615-799-5544, ext. 1; **bowiepark.org**
TRAIL SURFACE: Wood chips, pine needles, dirt	**LOCATION:** Fairview
HIKING TIME: 1.2 hours	**COMMENTS:** Trail may close after rainy periods. Call to confirm if trails are open.

own loop just trying to follow this one. Don't worry, though—it's hard to get really lost here, especially if you have a park map, which can be picked up online or at the trailhead.

From the parking area near the restrooms, walk around a wooden fence past the small playground toward the Lake Van Trail. A signed path leads downhill a short distance to access the actual Lake Van Trail. Take the wide path to the right, with the clear lake to your left, and cross over a wooden bridge. Relaxed anglers are sometimes seen sitting in chairs beside a pole, waiting for a bream to tug under the cork. Pass a couple of picnic shelters and curve around a small embayment of the lake. A wetland community has grown up in the margins that are neither lake nor land, and birdhouses have been nailed into lakeside trees.

The Lake Van Trail makes its way along the length of the impoundment. Notice cattails growing along the lake. Come to the lake dam and continue forward. Now you're on the Loblolly Loop (the Dome Trail goes to the right). True to the trail's name, tall loblolly trees along this path tower overhead, swaying with any gust of wind. Curve around on an old woods road and soon reach Upper Lake, which is visible through the trees to your left.

Circle Upper Lake and stay in pine woods. Don't be surprised to hear a woodpecker here. The dry ravine to your left is an old, failed dam. An unsigned side trail soon leaves right. Stay with the main old woods road and descend to another junction. Turn right here, looking for the sign that reads To Twin Lakes. Descend to step over an intermittent streambed, and then enter a small clearing on your right. This is deer country.

Before you know it, another lake appears—Lake Byrd. Walk across the dam of this lake and come to a picnic shelter at mile 1.4. This shelter overlooks the lake and makes a great midway picnic spot. Lake Anna is just a few steps down the trail beyond the picnic shelter. Here, the White Pine Trail leaves right. Stay left, though, and walk along the shore of Lake Anna 75 yards. Here, take an acute left away from the lake, not crossing the earthen dam. Soon look for the sign indicating Sycamore Springs. Turn right toward Sycamore Springs and descend into a moisture-loving hardwood forest that contrasts greatly with the piney woods encountered earlier. The tree canopy soon opens in a storm-damaged section before reaching the easily identifiable Sycamore Springs. This clear water source had been bricked and concreted in days gone by. Look for frogs in the water. Stick your hand in it—you'll find that the water is quite chilly. Come to another junction just past the spring. The Three Sisters–Perimeter Trail leaves right. Stay left, ascending a hill to reach the trailhead, and complete the loop.

Nearby Activities

This is more than a park with trails. Bowie Nature Park also has a nature center, several small lakes open to fishing, an elaborate playground for kids, and several picnic shelters. Consider making a day of it, and cook out.

GPS TRAILHEAD COORDINATES

N35° 58.237' W87° 8.313'

From Exit 182 on I-40, west of downtown Nashville, take TN 96 south 4.7 miles to TN 100 at Fairview. Turn right (west) on TN 100 and follow it 1.3 miles to Bowie Lake Road. Turn right on Bowie Lake Road and follow it 0.3 mile to the trailhead parking area on your right.

35 Meriwether Lewis Loop

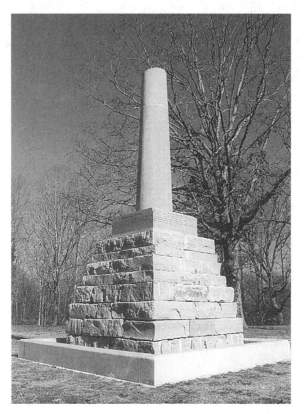

The monument to Meriwether Lewis rises on a stark winter day.

In Brief

This hike is centered on the Meriwether Lewis Monument, just off the Natchez Trace Parkway. Lewis died here in 1809, during his return trip to Washington, D.C., from St. Louis. The hike begins at Grinder's Stand, follows the historic Trace for a mile down to attractive Little Swan Creek, and eventually loops back to the monument area.

Description

This loop hike travels some very historic ground. It was at Grinder's Stand on the Natchez Trace, on October 11, 1809, where Meriwether Lewis died under circumstances that remain mysterious to this day. Following his famed expedition to the Pacific accompanied by William Clark, Lewis was appointed governor of Louisiana, which covered roughly 15

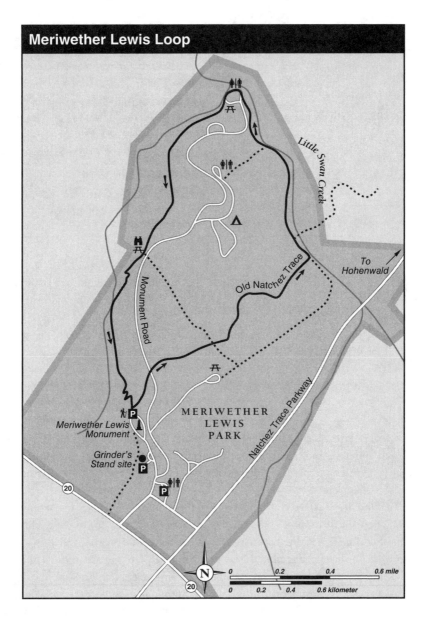

Meriwether Lewis Loop

million acres, essentially the extent of the Louisiana Purchase. The government did not honor some of his expenses for the expedition, so Lewis decided to return to Washington, D.C., to dispute them. He traveled south by water from St. Louis to the site of present-day Memphis, then headed east by land to avoid the British presence offshore, where he feared his expedition papers might be confiscated. Thus, he and a few companions found themselves on the Trace. Lewis arrived first at Grinder's Stand, where, according to Mrs. Grinder, "He seemed distraught all evening." Later that night, Mrs. Grinder heard shots

DISTANCE AND CONFIGURATION: 3.5-mile loop	**MAPS:** USGS *Gordonsburg;* at trailhead and at **tinyurl.com/lewismap;** Natchez Trace Parkway map at **tinyurl.com/natcheznash**
DIFFICULTY: Easy–moderate	
SCENERY: Ridge and streamside forest	
EXPOSURE: Mostly shady	**FACILITIES:** Restrooms, water at Meriwether Lewis campground during warm season, restrooms only in winter
TRAFFIC: Moderate	
TRAIL SURFACE: Dirt, rocks, leaves	**CONTACT:** 800-305-7417; **nps.gov/natr**
HIKING TIME: 2 hours	**LOCATION:** Hohenwald
ACCESS: No fees or permits required	**COMMENTS:** This loop is only one of several possible loop combinations at Meriwether Lewis Park.
PETS: On leash only	

and Lewis died the following day, at age 35, having already become one of America's greatest heroes. Whether he committed suicide or was murdered is one of our country's great historical uncertainties.

However, you can go to the very spot where Lewis died. A monument is nearby, and a stretch of the original Trace can be walked for a mile. Hikers then will pick up a foot trail that travels down the bluffs of Little Swan Creek, then up a feeder branch to make a loop. Start this hike at the trailhead log cabin, which has interesting historical exhibits about the Natchez Trace.

Take some time to absorb the information here. The stone outline of the Grinder's Stand cabin is near the log cabin, denoting the exact site where Lewis died. Head toward the stone monument, and read the inscriptions. The marble rectangles planted into the ground around the monument are graves of early settlers of Lewis County, giving rise to the name Pioneer Cemetery.

Pick up the original Trace at the far end of the monument. This is the actual start of the hike. Follow the Trace past a split cedar tree with two trunks. To your left, a hiker sign marks another trail; this is your return route. As you walk the Trace, consider how American history might have changed had Lewis walked the path you are on now, instead of having his journey cut short at Grinder's Stand. Considering his fame and popularity after his Corps of Discovery mission to the Pacific, he might have become president. The Meriwether Lewis Monument, a shaft extending skyward, is broken off at the top, symbolizing a life of potential greatness cut short for reasons unknown.

The original Trace soon crosses Monument Road, then passes another trail leading left, a loop shortcut. It becomes gullied as it descends to Peavyhouse Hollow and Little Swan Creek, where it meets a foot trail at mile 1. Turn left onto the foot trail; Little Swan Creek will be off to your right. Head downstream, soon climbing, as this side of the creek becomes a steep bluff. Reach a side trail leading left to the area campground. Continue in the Little Swan Creek valley, where views extend from the bluff. Soon you'll reach the picnic area. Walk across the picnic parking area, passing a copse of cedar trees at mile 1.7.

You'll enter the woods at a hiker trail sign with a couple of picnic tables off to your right. Now you're heading upstream along a noisy feeder branch of Little Swan Creek. The singletrack path works up the feeder-stream valley, circling in and out of side hollows. Turn away from the stream valley onto a hardwood ridgeline, reaching Monument Road at mile 2.7. Immediately turn away from the road, passing beneath a picnic table and overlook. Descend back into the feeder branch hollow by switchbacks and resume heading upstream in a fern-dotted flat, crossing the streambed twice in succession. Here the streambed is normally dry. Switchback out of the creek bed to emerge onto the original Trace near the Meriwether Lewis Monument at mile 3.5, ending the hike.

Nearby Activities

Meriwether Lewis Park has more than just hiking trails. The park roads and nearby Natchez Trace are good for bicycling. And there's a quiet, first-rate campground here. Nearby is the Buffalo River, which is great for paddling. Outfitters are located in nearby Hohenwald. Visit **nps.gov/natr** for more information.

GPS TRAILHEAD COORDINATES

N35° 30.693' W87° 27.667'

From Exit 46 on I-65, south of downtown Nashville, take US 412/TN 99 west 13.8 miles and then continue straight on US 43 for another 9.7 miles. Exit at Mount Joy Road, and head west for 7.6 miles. Make a slight left on Big Swan Creek Road, and in 3 miles, turn right on TN 20. In 5.8 miles turn right at the NATCHEZ TRACE PARKWAY/MERIWETHER LEWIS sign; then head to HISTORIC SITE AT MERIWETHER LEWIS MONUMENT. Park near the log cabin on the left.

---

36 Old Trace–Garrison Creek Loop

In Brief

Walk through time on this trek, picking up the original Natchez Trace, where travelers made their way from Natchez, Mississippi, to Nashville two centuries ago.

Description

The hike travels through varied environments on its journey from Burns Branch to Garrison Creek. The hike begins in quiet field and forest country on the Natchez Trace National Scenic Trail. The path heads up and down, winding in and out of small wooded coves, only to emerge onto the original Natchez Trace. It then makes a pleasant forest cruise on the longest section of Old Trace left in Tennessee, before taking a side path to a scenic overlook, where you can see the Garrison Creek valley and Middle Tennessee countryside.

Descend to Garrison Creek, picking up the Garrison Creek Loop Trail. Cross the clear stream twice before heading back toward the Old Trace. Here, the path takes an unexpected route, passing under the Natchez Trace Parkway via a modern tunnel built just for the hikers and equestrians who use this path. Climb a piney hillside before once again meeting the Old Trace, backtracking to the trailhead.

From the Burns Branch parking area, head north on the Natchez Trace National Scenic Trail toward Garrison Creek. Walk the margin of a field to enter a slice of woodland and cross a small feeder branch of Burns Branch, where a small pool is created by a flow from a culvert; look for fish in here. Keep north, paralleling a horse pasture in broken woods. Reach Davis Hollow Road at 0.6 mile. Cross the paved road and switchback up a hill grown over with hickory and oak trees.

Begin a pattern of dipping in and out of coves before reaching a clearing at mile 1.3. To your left is a picnic and parking area. Ahead is the beginning of a preserved section of the original Natchez Trace. It is hard to imagine all those who treaded this path before you. The Old Trace is much wider here than the path before and is more level, as it keeps forward on a high ridgeline. You'll soon reach a trail junction, and the Garrison Creek Loop Trail leaves left. This is your return route. Stay right, still following the Old Trace, keeping near the heavily wooded ridgetop. Steep ravines drop off on either side of the now rocky trail. Old wire fences parallel the path.

When you reach a second junction, leave the Old Trace and head left to the Garrison Creek Overlook. From here, you can see the valley to which you are headed. Make your way down to reach the Garrison Creek parking area at 3 miles. Here you'll find restrooms, a water spigot, and picnic tables. The main trail comes in from the right, just before reaching the building at the parking area.

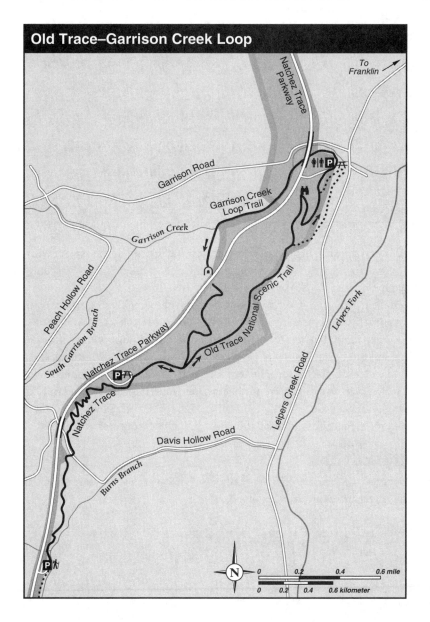

The trail seems to die out in the grassy fields. Fear not and keep downhill, reaching Garrison Creek and some streamside picnic tables. Now, keep upstream along the edge of the field beside the creek, contemplating a garrison of soldiers who camped along this stream as they built the Old Trace 200 years ago. Pass under the bridge of the parkway and watch for a dirt path, leaving right, to cross Garrison Creek. This is the continuation of the Garrison Creek Loop Trail. This is a wet crossing, meaning you aren't getting across unless you get your feet wet. Consider taking off your shoes and barefooting it across the

DISTANCE AND CONFIGURATION: 6.3-mile balloon	**PETS:** On leash only
	MAPS: USGS *Theta;* at **nps.gov/natt /upload/TennesseeTrail.pdf**
DIFFICULTY: Moderate	
SCENERY: Ridgetop and creekside forests	**FACILITIES:** Picnic tables at trailhead; restrooms, water at Garrison Creek, halfway through hike
EXPOSURE: Mostly shady	
TRAFFIC: Moderately busy on weekends	**CONTACT:** 800-305-7417; **nps.gov/natr**
TRAIL SURFACE: Dirt, rocks	**LOCATION:** Franklin
HIKING TIME: 3.5 hours	**COMMENTS:** The trail passes through a tunnel beneath the Natchez Trace Parkway.
ACCESS: No fees or permits required	

15 feet of normally shin-high water. As you ford, the clarity of the stream will surprise you. Back in their time, the soldiers who built the trail drank this water without purification or compunction. Those days are gone.

Keep upstream, in a sliver of woods between the creek and a field to your right. Enjoy an attractive and pleasant stroll before fording Garrison Creek at mile 3.8. Make a short but steep climb beyond the ford to reach the tunnel burrowing beneath the parkway. This short but exciting tunnel has an elevated sidewalk for pedestrians and a larger, lower, and wider way for horses. The trail then slabs the side of a ridgeline through piney woods, which give way to hardwoods before you reach the Old Trace at mile 4.8. Turn right here, following the Old Trace 0.2 mile. Keep backtracking south on the Natchez Trace National Scenic Trail to reach the Burns Branch parking area at mile 6.3.

Nearby Activities

The Natchez Trace Parkway offers not only scenic hiking but also scenic driving, picnicking, and insights into American history.

GPS TRAILHEAD COORDINATES
N35° 51.880' W87° 2.527'

From Exit 192 on I-40, west of downtown Nashville, take McCrory Lane 4.4 miles south to intersect TN 100. Turn right and immediately pick up the Natchez Trace Parkway. Head south on the parkway 16.2 miles to the Burns Branch parking area on your left. The Natchez Trace National Scenic Trail heads in both directions. Take the scenic trail north, heading toward Garrison Creek.

37 Perimeter Trail

In Brief

Operated by the town of Fairview, Bowie Nature Park traverses mildly rolling Middle Tennessee forestland not usually slated for preservation. The Bowie sisters, longtime Fairview residents, rehabilitated this cut-over, burned-over, and eroded land, then deeded it to the town of Fairview. What remains today is an attractive forest with trees of differing ages, cut by clear creeks forming small valleys. The distance is the most challenging aspect of the hike.

Description

Parks historically have been created and preserved in large part due to the exceptional beauty of the land's physical features. As far as beauty, Bowie Nature Park is in a league of its own. Land like Bowie Nature Park is typically used for farmland or pastureland, or is otherwise developed. In the past, this land was agriculturally mismanaged. But thanks to Evangeline Bowie and her two sisters, it was rehabilitated and deeded to the city of Fairview, which now runs the property as a park.

The Perimeter Trail, which makes a loop along the edge of the 800-acre park, is great for hikers who want to extend their trips but not get on something too tough. Though you may not always get a feel of being in the wild, the fields and woods of the park provide an ideal habitat for wildlife. The trail is a mixture of old woods roads and singletrack trail. Quiet hikers in early mornings and evenings are likely to spot deer that roam the park. Since much of the path is not canopied, I recommend hiking here during fall, winter, and spring—summer can be hot. Be aware that the trail may be closed after heavy rains; call ahead to make sure it's open. As a footnote, the trail is open not only to hikers but also to mountain bikers. I have never had a problem with them as they pedal the path, but you should listen for them on weekend hikes.

To start the Perimeter Trail, leave the trailhead and parking area behind and head west toward the Tennessee Valley Authority (TVA) electric line, keeping downhill to reach the Sycamore Springs Trail on the far side of the power line. Descend along an old road to soon reach a trail junction. Veer left onto the red-blazed Three Sisters–Perimeter Trail, soon entering thicker woods to reach Little Turnbull Creek at 0.5 mile. Work away from the creek in mixed hardwoods with many dogwoods, and again come to the TVA line. Veer left and cruise along the line 0.3 mile before reentering pine and oak woods with a broken canopy. The trail turns northwest and passes near Hidden Hollow Creek before reaching an old cemetery at mile 2.1. One grave is marked, but the rest are simply fieldstones languishing under the shade of dogwood trees.

Continue downhill and reach Little Turnbull Creek, a clear, rock-bottomed stream that's backed by stone bluffs. The creek can be dry-footed most of the year. A foot trail

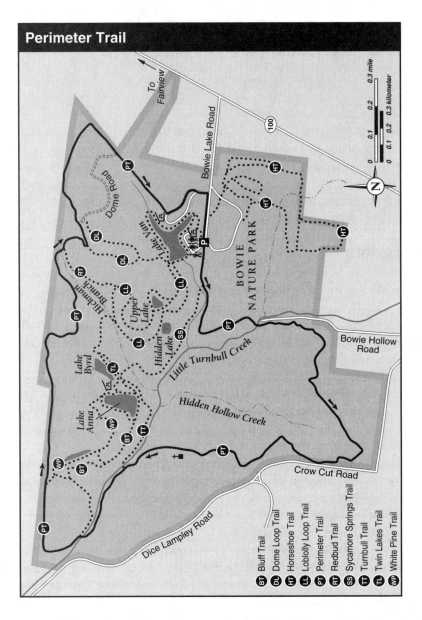

Perimeter Trail

heads upstream from the crossing. The Perimeter Trail briefly keeps downstream before climbing away from the watercourse and heading due east along the park border, intersecting the White Pine Trail. Continue as the trail moves through small valleys of mixed hardwoods and piney hills.

At mile 4, the Dome Trail leaves right, and the Perimeter Trail makes a U-turn left, soon passing another branch of the Dome Trail. Stay in broken woods before passing under the TVA line. Continue south to emerge at Bowie Lake Road at mile 4.9. Turn right on Bowie Lake Road and walk through the parking area to complete the loop.

DISTANCE AND CONFIGURATION: 5.1-mile loop	**ACCESS:** No fees or permits required; daily, sunrise–sunset
DIFFICULTY: Moderate	**PETS:** On leash only
SCENERY: Woodlands, small streamsheds	**MAPS:** USGS *Craigfield*; at **bowiepark.org**
EXPOSURE: Part sun, part shade	**FACILITIES:** Water spigot, restrooms, picnic area
TRAFFIC: Very little during the week, some trail users on weekends	**CONTACT:** 615-799-5544, ext. 1; **bowiepark.org**
TRAIL SURFACE: Dirt	**LOCATION:** Fairview
HIKING TIME: 2.5 hours	**COMMENTS:** Trail may close after rainy periods. Call to confirm if trails are open.

Nearby Activities

This is more than a park with trails. Bowie Nature Park also has a nature center, several small lakes open to fishing, an elaborate playground for kids, and several picnic shelters. Consider making a day of it, and cook out.

GPS TRAILHEAD COORDINATES

N35° 58.237' W87° 8.313'

From Exit 182 on I-40, west of downtown Nashville, take TN 96 south 4.7 miles to TN 100 at Fairview. Turn right (west) on TN 100 and follow it 1.3 miles to Bowie Lake Road. Turn right on Bowie Lake Road and follow it 0.3 mile to the trailhead parking area on your right.

SOUTHEAST

INCLUDING BRENTWOOD, MURFREESBORO, AND SMYRNA

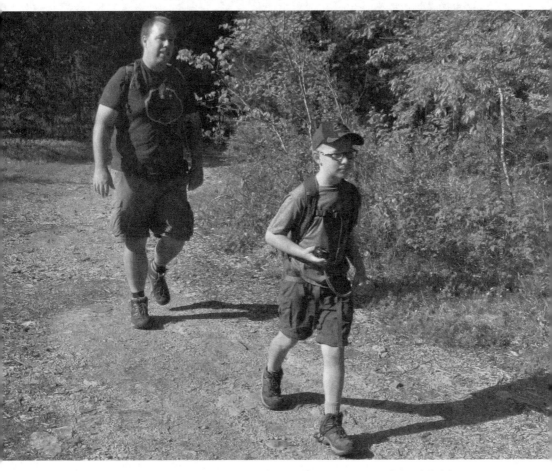

*Avid hikers Carl and Michael Nelson on the Stones River National Battlefield Loop
(see page 181)*

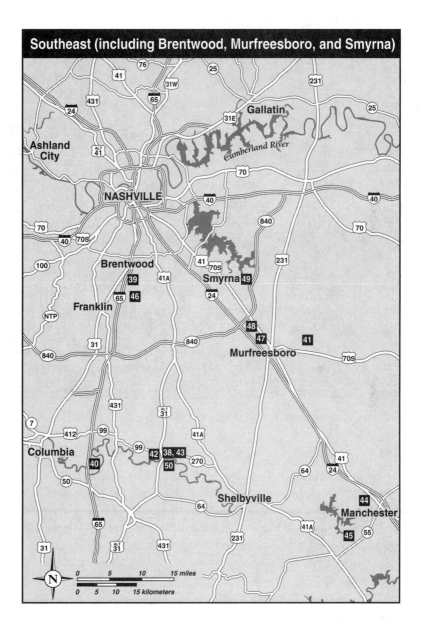

Southeast (including Brentwood, Murfreesboro, and Smyrna)

38 Adeline Wilhoite River Trail

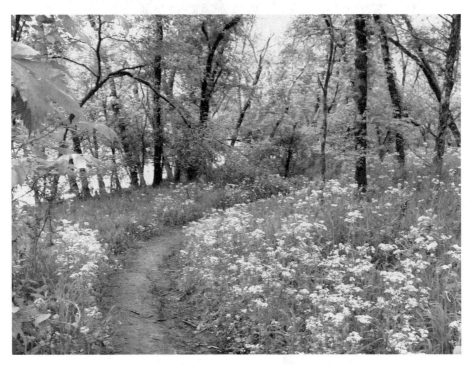

The River Trail adorned in flowers during springtime

In Brief

This hike journeys along Duck River, a state scenic waterway, cruising through bottom-lands and presenting aquatic panoramas before climbing to a bluff, where an observation tower overlooks restored native grassland. From there, make a loop through hardwood forests and cedar glades. Additionally, this hike has a backcountry campsite along the way, availing the possibility of backpacking during the trek.

Description

Henry Horton State Park has long been a go-to recreation destination for greater Nash-ville. Adeline Wilhoite River Trail adds another reason to come here. Along this path you will get to stride the shore of Duck River, maybe taking a side trip to one of the rock out-crops that stand along the Tennessee state scenic river. Or maybe you will enjoy walking the richly vegetated bottomlands rife with wildflowers in spring. Or maybe you will relish

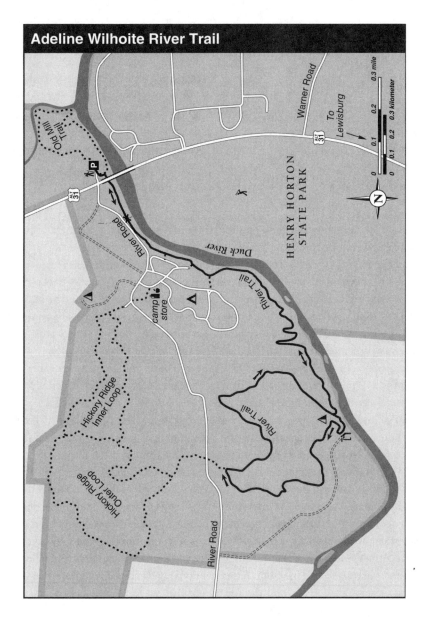

climbing the observation tower, built into a large tree that watches over restored grassland, a place where deer are often seen in the morning and evening. Or maybe you will
want to walk through cedar glades, the unique yet imperiled ecosystem found in Middle
Tennessee. Or maybe you will appreciate wandering amid former farmland turned forest
that still harbors evidence of its agricultural past. Or maybe you will simply want to strap
on your backpack and head to the trail's backcountry campsite situated on a bluff above

DISTANCE AND CONFIGURATION: 4.1-mile balloon	**ACCESS:** No fees or permits required
DIFFICULTY: Moderate	**PETS:** On leash only
SCENERY: River views, cedar glades	**MAPS:** USGS *Farmington;* at **tnstate parks.com/parks/about/henry-horton**
EXPOSURE: Mostly shady	**FACILITIES:** Campground nearby, picnic area, restrooms across river
TRAFFIC: Busy on nice-weather weekends	**CONTACT:** 931-364-2222; **tnstateparks .com/parks/about/henry-horton**
TRAIL SURFACE: Natural	**LOCATION:** Chapel Hill
HIKING TIME: 2 hours	

Duck River. No matter your primary reason, this walkway will uphold the tradition of fine recreation at Henry Horton State Park.

River Trail and Old Mill Trail both leave from the same trailhead. However, River Trail splits right and heads under the US 31A Bridge and shortly joins an old roadbed running parallel with the river. Below you, the green Duck River flows west, the same direction you are hiking, bordered by rock outcrops that make for popular fishing spots. Spur trails lead down to these locales. Ash and sycamore shade the path. At 0.2 mile, cross an intermittent streambed on a wooden bridge, just below a small, seasonal waterfall. Quickly pass a second bridge. At 0.4 mile, a spur trail heads right to the park campground, near campsite 10. Keep straight with River Trail, gaining views of Duck River while hiking moist flats that can be a bit muddy after rains.

At 0.9 mile, River Trail turns away from the river and works around a small limestone-lined tributary, then curves around a second intermittent stream before returning alongside the river. Hickory and walnut are prevalent here. At 1.1 miles, the trail runs alongside an island in Duck River. The channel is just below you. Even though you are well above the river, look for evidence of flooding during high-water events, such as brush and limbs piled on the upstream sides of trees. It is hard to imagine the Duck getting this high, but it periodically does. Come to the loop portion of the hike at 1.3 miles. Keep straight here, crossing a spring then turning away from the river. Here, you will come alongside a wetland prairie, a 35-acre former field the park has restored to native grasses through prescribed fire. Reach a wildlife observation deck built into a tree overlooking the meadow. Climb the deck and give the prairie a gander. Beyond the tower, climb a hill to reach a backcountry campground. Multiple campsites are situated in level woods, each with a tent pad and fire ring. You must register in advance to reserve the campsite. The hike remains level here as you navigate rocky woods. This area was once farmland and you will be skirting off and on old farm roads, dancing between old wire fences, metal relics and other evidence of the agricultural past, now cloaked in cedars and hardwoods. While most of Middle Tennessee is moving from forest to urbanity, this neck of the woods is going the opposite way.

Come to a junction at 2 miles. Here, a connector trail heads left, north, to Hickory Ridge Loop. However, River Trail turns right, winding in and out of cedar glades and old fields mixed with woods. The walking is easy, so you can focus on looking for more

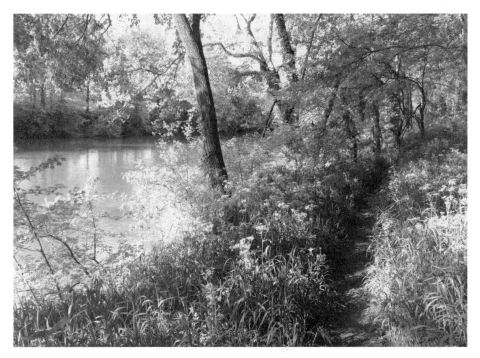

Hike through riverside bottomlands on this trail adventure.

agricultural relics—and wildlife, as this blend of tree and meadow makes for attractive habitat. Expect to see deer and/or wild turkeys. At 2.4 miles, River Trail curves south then crosses a normally dry streambed and meanders richly wooded bottomland to finish the loop portion of the trail at 2.8 miles. From here it is a 1.3-mile backtrack to the trailhead.

Nearby Activities

Henry Horton State Park has a developed campground with water and electricity, a primitive tent campground, and other amenities such as a golf course, a lodge, a restaurant, and even a trap- and skeet-shooting range.

GPS TRAILHEAD COORDINATES

N35° 35.612' W86° 41.755'

From Exit 46 on I-65, south of Nashville, head east on TN 99 for 4 miles to US 431. Turn right (south), and in 0.8 mile, continue east on TN 99 for another 7.4 miles to US 31 Alternate. Turn right on US 31A and follow it south 0.5 mile to Henry Horton State Park. Look left for a parking area just before US 31A bridges Duck River. This left turn is just across from the right turn into the state park campground.

39 Brenthaven Bikeway Connector

In Brief

This greenway connects two parks operated by the city of Brentwood: River Park and Crockett Park. The trail traverses an attractive wooded corridor along Little Harpeth River, which makes it one of the most attractive greenways in metro Nashville.

Description

I heard about this greenway from a friend of a friend. As it turns out, this connector trail between River Park to the north and Crockett Park to the south is popular with Brentwood residents—walkers, runners, and bicyclists alike. Similar to many areas of metro Nashville, the city of Brentwood is growing rapidly. However, this greenway and the adjacent parks are examples of the city planning and growing its recreational needs along with the increased population. A fine library is just across the street from the north trailhead, River Park. When designing this library, the city planners included ample green space along with extensions of the greenway, integrating the latter into the overall design rather than adding it as an afterthought.

Luckily for us, the city had some good natural terrain to work with. It so happens that the scenic Little Harpeth River flows through this section of Brentwood, and this river corridor made for a likely and available slice of land on which to put a greenway. Little Harpeth River is longer than you may imagine. It actually drains 895 square miles of land, mostly in Williamson County. Soldiers from North Carolina, who received land grants for their efforts during the Revolutionary War, first settled the Brentwood area. Many plantations were in the area by the time of the Civil War. During the war, the area was pilfered of its crops and farm animals, and the homes were used as makeshift hospitals. The area languished after the Civil War but grew again after the coming of I-65 in the 1960s. It has since become a major bedroom community of Nashville.

Little Harpeth River flows adjacent to the River Park parking area. Look for the greenway bridge and begin your walk. Span Little Harpeth River and turn south; the YMCA is off to your left. Sycamores shade Little Harpeth River, which flows in riffles, pools, and occasional rocky shoals. During winter, houses are visible through the trees. Occasionally, black-painted wooden fences, like those seen at horse farms, border the trail. Williamson County was horse country before suburbanization made its way down here, and its residents still pride themselves on this equestrian association. Plenty of horse farms still exist in rural sections of the county.

At 0.5 mile, the canopy opens overhead. A partially wooded wetland lies to the left of the trail, and to your right Little Harpeth River has widened as it flows over a limestone slab

148

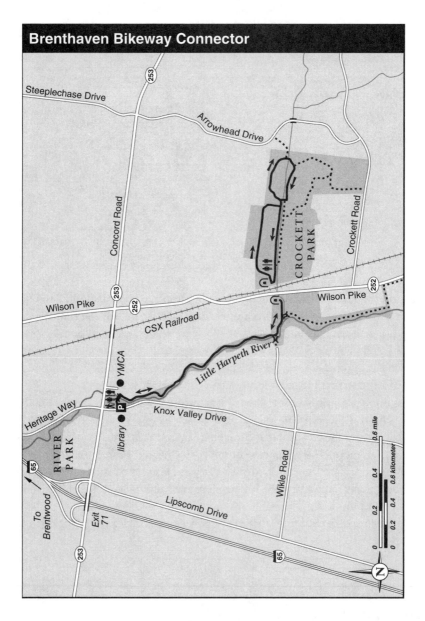

Brenthaven Bikeway Connector

cutting across the watercourse. Little Harpeth had another name long ago, one that would excite anglers. In 1768 Thomas Hutchins named the river Fish Creek because he must have eaten a few meals out of this clear-green watercourse. By the 1780s the name Harpeth began appearing on maps. It was likely derived from Big Harp and Little Harp, two highwaymen whose ilk was common in this era when Middle Tennessee was sparsely populated. Such bandits would typically lie in wait for unsuspecting travelers and rob them.

DISTANCE AND CONFIGURATION: 2.4-mile out-and-back	**MAPS:** USGS *Franklin;* at **tinyurl.com /brenthavenmap**
DIFFICULTY: Easy	**FACILITIES:** Restrooms, water at Crockett Park
SCENERY: Riparian forests, stream	
EXPOSURE: Partly shady	**CONTACT:** 615-371-0080; **brentwood -tn.org/index.aspx?page=144**
TRAFFIC: Busy	**LOCATION:** Brentwood
TRAIL SURFACE: Asphalt	**COMMENTS:** The greenway is extended on both ends, adding walking distance opportunities. River Park has basketball courts. The Brentwood Library is just across the street from River Park. And Crockett Park has tennis courts, ball fields, and picnic shelters.
HIKING TIME: 1.4 hours	
ACCESS: No fees or permits required; Crockett Park: daily, 8 a.m.–10 p.m.; River Park: daily, sunrise–sunset	
PETS: On leash only	

Ahead is a massive trailside oak tree with a trunk so wide it would easily take two people together to wrap their arms around the giant. At mile 1, the trail splits. To the right, a bridge leads over Little Harpeth River to Wikle Road and houses; this is also where the Boiling Springs/Ravenwood Greenway heads south for miles, then turns east and north back up to Crockett Road. The main path curves left, now alongside a feeder branch of Little Harpeth River. A large open field is beside the trail.

Pass through a pair of tunnels, the first tunnel passing beneath Wilson Road and the second beneath CSX Railroad tracks. At mile 1.2, just beyond the tracks, you'll reach Crockett Park and the end of this section of greenway. This large park has tennis courts, ball fields, and more. The greenway continues in Crockett Park, making a pair of small loops. And a side path leads to Arrowhead Drive. This section is not nearly as scenic as the portion along Little Harpeth. It does, however, offer added distance for increased exercise opportunities.

The trail extends west from River Park as well, entering Concord Park and forming two loops.

GPS TRAILHEAD COORDINATES

N35° 59.758' W86° 47.258'

From Exit 71 on I-65, south of downtown Nashville, take TN 253/Concord Road east 0.5 mile to Knox Valley Drive. Turn right on Knox Valley Drive and follow it just a short distance to River Park, on your left. Start this section of the greenway by crossing the bridge over Little Harpeth River near the basketball courts.

40 Cheeks Bend Bluff View Trail

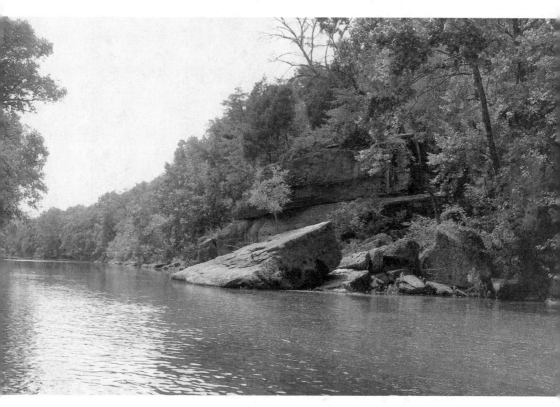

View of the Duck River near Cheeks Bend

In Brief

Explore this special Tennessee State Natural Areas holding. Cheeks Bend is part of the 2,135-acre Duck River State Natural Area Complex. The trail travels along a bluff overlooking Duck River and includes a special surprise—a cave near the river at the base of the bluff.

Description

This trail goes by a cave with a 100-foot-or-so passage—now closed to combat white-nose syndrome, a bat disease not communicable to humans—that leads from a river bluff

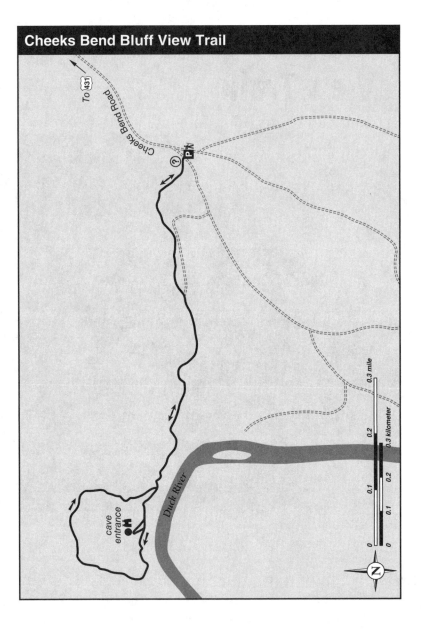

overlooking Duck River to the base of the same bluff. At least you will be able to check out the cave entrance. Cheeks Bend Vista Trail starts on the west side of the road. Begin following a singletrack path into the woods to reach a trailside kiosk showing the trail and giving information about the Duck River Complex. This complex is an agglomeration of six separate natural areas collectively within the Yanahli Wildlife Management Area. All are located in the Duck River basin and include Columbia Glade, Sowell Mill, Rummage

DISTANCE AND CONFIGURATION: 1.8-mile balloon	**ACCESS:** No fees or permits required
DIFFICULTY: Easy	**PETS:** On leash only
SCENERY: River bluff, cedar woods, cave, riverside	**MAPS:** USGS *Glendale;* at **tinyurl.com /cheeksbend**
EXPOSURE: Mostly shady	**FACILITIES:** None
TRAFFIC: Not much	**CONTACT:** 615-781-6500; **tinyurl.com /duckrivercomplex**
TRAIL SURFACE: Rocks, dirt	
HIKING TIME: 1 hour	**LOCATION:** Columbia

Cave, Howard Bridge Glades, and Moore Lane, in addition to Cheeks Bend. This part of Duck River is significant, as 13 of the 30 miles of the state scenic-river portion of the Duck are located here.

The blue-blazed track descends into oak–hickory–cedar woods, picking up an old roadbed. Here, the path makes an abrupt left turn, leaving the roadbed to cross a wet-weather branch. It then continues downhill, only to recross the branch just above a multi-tiered waterfall that likely won't fall at all in late summer and autumn. Duck River is visible through the trees in the winter.

Curve around to cross another wet-weather branch, and on your left you'll see Duck River, which is a good 30 feet below the trail but can be accessed here. Work your way down to reach some riverside rock outcrops that make for ideal sunning spots. Turtles know these are good sunning spots too; you'll see them splashing into the river as you head down. This isn't the ideal swimming hole, though, as the river is strongly sweeping around the bend here.

The path now ascends among pale rock outcrops as it works to the top of a bluff. Reach the loop portion of the trail at 0.6 mile. Continue, still stairstepping up the bluff, with obscured views of the river below. Ferns and mosses offer green contrast to the white outcrops, and cedars cling to shallow soils on the bluff. Reach the edge of the bluff, and you can look downriver southwest toward I-65, which isn't visible but is audible.

The bluff levels off and reaches a junction. Watch carefully here for a cedar tree banded with both blue and red stripes. To reach the cave, turn right here and follow the red blazes away from the river and down to a cave entrance that's not visible from where you stand. The cave entrance is nearly square and big enough for a man to stand in. It is now closed to visitors, but you can still look and see the light penetrating the cave from the other opening.

Return to the main trail and keep along the bluff, where you can see fields and woods across the river. At 0.8 mile, the trail turns away from the river, passing through a good spring-wildflower area before stairstepping over more outcrops to reach a high point. From there, work downhill while passing linear sinks. Complete the loop portion of the hike at 1.2 miles, and then backtrack to the trailhead.

Nearby Activities

Paddling Duck River lends a different perspective to this beautiful valley. River Rat's canoe operation is located at the intersection of TN 99 and US 431, which you will pass on the way to Cheeks Bend. (There are two intersections of US 431 and TN 99; River Rat's is at the more southerly one.) Offering canoe rentals and shuttles on Duck River, they can be reached at 931-381-2278 or **riverratcanoe.com.**

GPS TRAILHEAD COORDINATES

N35° 34.063' W86° 53.100'

From Exit 46 on I-65, take TN 99/Bear Creek Pike east 4 miles to US 431. Turn right, and take US 431 5.7 miles south to reach Jordan Road. Turn right on Jordan Road (the left turn at this intersection is Wiles Lane). Follow Jordan Road 2.5 miles west, crossing Duck River (along the way, Jordan Road becomes Sowell Mill Pike). In another 0.8 mile after crossing the river, watch for the left turn onto gravel Cheeks Bend Road. Follow Cheeks Bend Road 0.9 mile to the trailhead.

41 Flat Rock Cedar Glades and Barrens Hike

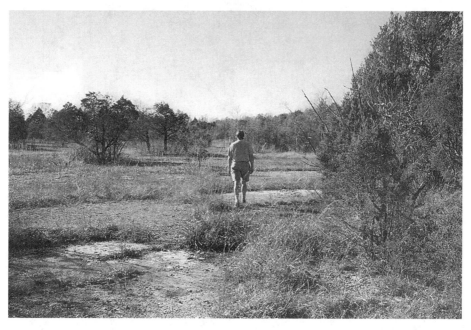

A hiker crosses an open cedar glade.

In Brief

This special area, bought and preserved by the Nature Conservancy in conjunction with the state of Tennessee, has become more special with the expansion of its trail system. Flat Rock is one of the largest remaining intact cedar glades. The expanded loop wanders among cedar woods and along barren rock glades, grassy glades, and hardwood forest. Along the way it passes a clear, alluring spring and a sinkhole, where a creek flows into it and disappears underground.

Description

Flat Rock is one of Tennessee's largest intact cedar glade preserves, protecting 600 acres of the Southeast's rarest habitats. Working in conjunction with the Tennessee State Natural Areas Program, the Nature Conservancy played a large role in protecting this land, specifically known as a limestone-outcrop glade. Barren in appearance, this habitat is home to very rare plants. One flower in particular, Pyne's ground plum, is found here and at only

Flat Rock Cedar Glades and Barrens Hike

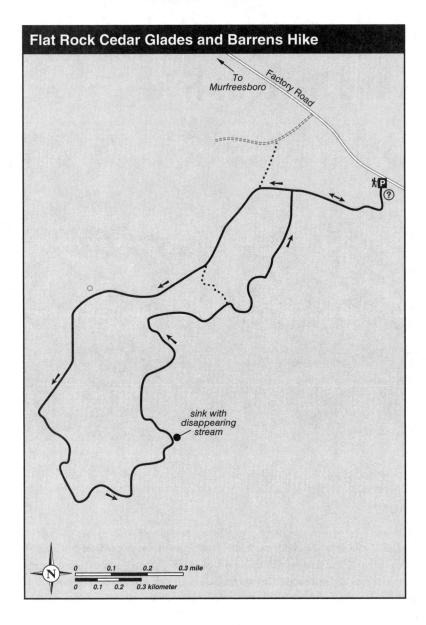

To Murfreesboro

Factory Road

sink with
disappearing
stream

0   0.1   0.2   0.3 mile

0   0.1   0.2   0.3 kilometer

N

three other known sites in the world. Pyne's ground plum was once thought to be extinct. Within this preserve are other rare plants, such as purple prairie clover and the sunnybell lily. As with other landscapes of this type, sinks, caves, and water seeps dot the seemingly dry landscape. This underground flow of water plays a large role in shaping the plants and animals that thrive in this harsh-looking country. Above ground, wet-weather washes harbor endangered plant species such as Boykin's milkwort.

DISTANCE AND CONFIGURATION: 3.4-mile balloon	**ACCESS:** No fees or permits required
	PETS: On leash only
DIFFICULTY: Moderate	**MAPS:** USGS *Dillton;* at **tinyurl.com/flatrocksna**
SCENERY: Cedar and hardwood forest, large cedar barrens	
	FACILITIES: None
EXPOSURE: Half shady, half sunny	**CONTACT:** 615-532-0431; **tinyurl.com/flatrocksna**
TRAFFIC: You will have the trail to yourself.	
	LOCATION: Murfreesboro
TRAIL SURFACE: Rocks, dirt	**COMMENTS:** This may be the best-preserved cedar glade environment in Middle Tennessee.
HIKING TIME: 2 hours	

The Nature Conservancy invested in this site not only because of Pyne's ground plum and the other rare plants but also because man's impact on the site was minimal. You will see evidence of past use here, but it doesn't detract from this great hike.

The expanded path, traveling through the preserve, is one of Middle Tennessee's newer trails. Leave the parking area, shortly passing a plaque commemorating the preservation of the locale. Pass a trailside kiosk with trail maps, and then enter a cedar thicket. The trail is marked by blue blazes, though you will also see occasional white blazes and—more important—posts tipped in blue with arrows pointing in the correct direction. Follow these posts carefully, as the path heads through many open glades. At 0.1 mile, turn right, passing behind a nearby residence. Pick up a rocky woods road along a fence line.

At 0.3 mile, you'll reach a junction; to your left is your return route. Continue forward here, climbing a hill. Flat Rock Preserve does have vertical variation, as evidenced by the views of oak-cloaked hills in the distance from the wide-open glade. Veer left onto an old farm road, and at 0.6 mile reach a trail junction. Here, the old loop keeps forward, but the newer, blue-blazed loop turns right and heads uphill through woods, passing an old junk pile before reaching a spring at 1 mile. Watch as the water passes beneath the trail via a small culvert. The clear spring is to your right and emerges from a round pool about 8 feet in diameter. You can be sure that early settlers took note of this spring.

The trail continues ascending, with a rocky hill to the right, and traces an old roadbed until 1.3 miles, where it turns left and descends. Look left in the woods for the dam of an old farm pond. Along the hike you may notice where young cedars have been cut down. This is part of the glade-restoration process, which also uses prescribed burns.

At 1.5 miles, the trail winds through an open glade where old poles are stacked. The path winds in and out of small glades before reaching an area with many yucca plants at 1.9 miles. Then the trail enters a dense cedar copse and reaches a significant sinkhole at 2 miles. Here, a stream flows into the sink, briefly running in the hole before disappearing into the ground. This is indicative of the area's karst topography, which is a fancy word for holey eroded ground where water and rock interplay beneath the surface, resulting in both springs and sinks. You will undoubtedly also notice trash in the sink. Historically, settlers in glade-and-sink country placed farm debris and trash in the depressions to fill them up and stop the sinking of water from the surface. Even more elementary, the nature-made holes were good dumps. The result was tainted water supplies wherever the water reemerged from the sink. Today, people are more aware of the interrelationship of land and water, and this practice is on the wane.

The trail continues through the best of what Flat Rock has to offer, but watch carefully as the trail goes where you think it won't—or shouldn't. At 2.7 miles, you'll reach the old inner loop in a large gravelly glade. At first glance, the area looks like a parking lot grown over with weeds. But these weed-looking plants are actually some of the life that is so rare in this rare habitat. The flowers that grow in this barren area are best observed mid-August–mid-September, though other good wildflower displays are mid-April–mid-May.

This spot is one large gravel glade, an important reason the Nature Conservancy purchased this tract. Areas known as post-oak barrens also support native grasses and endangered flowers, such as slender blazing star. The trail continues northeast, winding among more glades before completing the loop portion of the hike at 3.1 miles. Turn right here and backtrack to the trailhead.

Nearby Activities

Consider combining this excursion with a trip on the Stones River Greenway of Murfreesboro or a visit to Stones River National Battlefield. Both are nearby and detailed in this book (see pages 178 and 181).

GPS TRAILHEAD COORDINATES

N35° 51.428' W86° 17.557'

From Exit 78B on I-24, southeast of downtown Nashville, take TN 96 East 3.1 miles to Clark Boulevard. Turn right on East Clark Boulevard and follow it 1.4 miles to Greenland Drive. Turn left on Greenland Drive as it turns into Halls Hill Pike, traveling a total of 4.1 miles to Factory Road. Turn right on Factory Road and follow it 1 mile to the parking area for the preserve, which will be on your right. Watch carefully for the brown sign indicating the preserve, as it is easily missed.

42 Hickory Ridge Trail

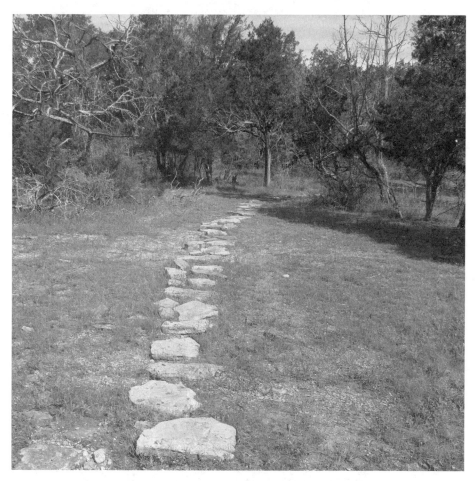

Stepping-stones lead hikers through a trailside clearing.

In Brief

This hike explores incredible sinkholes, stony rock gardens, and cedar glades while mixing in some history. You will first traverse a dense concentration of sinkholes scattered amid crazy rock gardens, then walk rich woods to find an Indian marker tree. Curve through formerly settled land to find an old rocked-in spring, important for early settlers, before returning to sinkhole-rich rolling terrain, where a few hills add vertical variation to the hike.

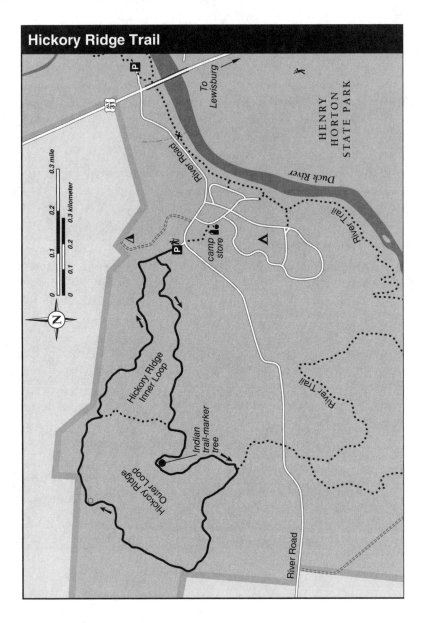

Description

Hickory Ridge Trail is an easy loop walk for those staying at the Henry Horton State Park campground, as a leg of it starts at the camp store. This trail is also convenient for those staying in the drive-up primitive campground at the park. The path was formerly shorter, but an outer loop was added to the Hickory Ridge Trail in 2014. This additional circuit not only adds mileage to the hike but also explores more terrain, including cedar glades, refreshing woods, and settler sites, including a spring rocked in and used by the earliest

DISTANCE AND CONFIGURATION: 2.3-mile loop	**ACCESS:** No fees or permits required
DIFFICULTY: Easy–moderate	**PETS:** On leash only
SCENERY: Sinkholes, rock gardens, settler evidence	**MAPS:** USGS *Farmington;* at **tnstate parks.com/parks/about/henry-horton**
EXPOSURE: Mostly shady	**FACILITIES:** Campground and camp store nearby, picnic area, restrooms across river
TRAFFIC: Busy when state park campground is full	**CONTACT:** 931-364-2222; **tnstateparks .com/parks/about/henry-horton**
TRAIL SURFACE: Natural	
HIKING TIME: 1.5 hours	**LOCATION:** Chapel Hill

settlers in the Duck River basin. Yet you will see something perhaps even older, the American Indian trail-marker tree. Here, an oak was bent over and shaped to form a directional arrow to help aboriginal Tennesseans find their way. What this trail-marker tree led to or from has been lost to time. Although trees sometimes end up with this shape accidentally due to storms or other trees falling on them, we know this is a marker tree; damaged trees have obvious scars on them, while trail-marker trees were shaped and intended to continue living in an altered form.

Trail-marker trees were first bent over in the desired direction, then tied to the ground with a vine, after which the tree began growing back toward the sky. This formed an easily identifiable horizontal trunk, creating the directional marker. This particular trail-marker tree is mature and stands out in the forest.

Speaking of trees, shagbark hickories thrive in the rocky woods protected by this part of Henry Horton State Park. With loose-plated bark sloughing off the main trunk, shagbark hickories look like what their name implies, shaggy-haired humans who could use a trim. The loose bark plates run vertically up the trunk of the tree.

Found all over the Volunteer State, shagbark hickories once were an important food source for aboriginal Tennesseans, who sought out their surprisingly sweet nuts. The nuts were used by American pioneers much as you would use a pecan. However, attempts at commercial propagation of the shagbark hickory have been unsuccessful. In the wild, nut production varies wildly year to year. The thinner shell and greater nutmeat make shagbark hickory nuts an attractive choice. Indians even made hickory nut soup. They also broke the nuts, collected the meat, and pounded them down to release oils. They would then form the meat into balls, with the oil keeping the pulverized acorns intact. These "nutballs" were an ideal way to store the food for later use, since they could be quickly and easily eaten, as opposed to breaking the shells and removing the meat. The best time to collect the nuts was soon after the oak acorns fell and before the first frost of autumn. Mammals and birds competed with the Indians in getting to the sought-after hickory nuts, especially when the shagbark's nut production was down.

Hickory Ridge Trail leaves the parking area and runs parallel to the primitive campground. Shortly split left and join what is now known as the Inner Loop. Begin a crash course into and through rocky-to-the-extreme woods pocked with a maze of sinkholes. Scattered cedar glades enhance the biodiversity. The path remains level in shagbark hickory–laden flatwoods. At 0.5 mile, pass the trail leading right to make the Inner Loop. Keep straight, joining the Outer Loop, and soon circle by the aforementioned Indian trail-marker tree. The hike enters a transitional area, with more open cedar glades. At 0.9 mile, Hickory Ridge Trail meets a connector trail leading left to Adeline Wilhoite River Trail. Keep straight here, drifting through more cedar glades, the path lined in flat stones through the clearings. Bridge an intermittent streambed at 1.2 miles. Ahead, the trail traverses more cedar glades and through woods. At 1.5 miles, after a descent, pass the rocked-in spring on your right. You can rest assured a homesite was nearby; however, the dense woods obscure it. Climb away from the spring, passing a showcase of sinkholes, a geological wonderment giving clues to the complicated underground plumbing system of Middle Tennessee.

At 1.8 miles, return to the Inner Loop. Split left here, wandering among hills before reentering the über-rocky sinkhole area. At 2.2 miles, come within sight of the primitive campground. Shortly complete the loop and backtrack to the trailhead. If you are thirsty, stop at the camp store for a drink and a treat. You earned it.

Nearby Activities

Henry Horton State Park has a developed campground with water and electricity, a primitive tent campground, and other amenities such as a golf course, a lodge, a restaurant, and even a trap- and skeet-shooting range.

GPS TRAILHEAD COORDINATES

N35° 35.525' W86° 42.197'

From Exit 46 on I-65, south of Nashville, head east on TN 99 for 4 miles to US 431. Turn right (south), and in 0.8 mile, continue east on TN 99 for another 7.4 miles to US 31 Alternate. Turn right on US 31A and follow it south 0.5 mile to Henry Horton State Park. Just before US 31A bridges Duck River, take the right turn toward the state park campground on River Road and follow it 0.3 mile to the trailhead, just after the right turn into the Primitive Campground.

43 Old Mill Trail

In Brief

Old Mill Trail traverses the most historic parcel of Henry Horton State Park. The path loops along the scenic Duck River through an area that was once the thriving hamlet of Wilhoites Mill. Experience firsthand the fading of history, as second-growth woods slowly camouflage the remains of a community that thrived in the 1800s.

Description

The Old Mill hike is a walk into history, heading through a community once known as Wilhoites Mill. This first white settlement in the Duck River Valley began in the late 1700s. Later, Andrew Jackson himself crossed the river here while establishing a road, at what was then known as Fishing Ford, on the way to the Battle of New Orleans. Later, a stage line followed Jackson's road, and a log inn was built where the state park inn now stands. In the 1820s, the first bridge was built over Duck River at this location. This bridge and many others, including a covered bridge erected in 1838 (you can still see its rock piers), were subsequently built and swept away by floods. Around 1845, Addie Wilhoite bought the log inn. Her son John built a mill, grinding corn and grain along Duck River. It was around this mill that the community of Wilhoites Mill grew. John Wilhoite married and had a daughter who married Henry Horton, later a US senator and the governor of Tennessee from 1927 to 1933. Henry Horton returned to his home on Duck River, but he died just one year after ending his term as governor. His son John operated the mill until 1959, when the site was purchased by the state of Tennessee for the establishment of the state park you see today.

Leave the parking area and walk toward the bridge, descending on a path of wood chips. Immediately to your left is a large iron wheel, which was turned by a long belt, connected to turbines located on the river. This setup kept most of the mill on higher ground, as the original mill had been wiped out in a 1902 flood during which Duck River rose 47 feet in 11 hours. Just below here the Adeline Wilhoite River Trail leaves right and heads under the road bridge and downstream along the river. This hike, however, turns left, upriver. Keep walking down to the water, and on its bank you'll see the rock-filled cedar cribs that held the turbines. A low dam diverted water through the turbines that drove the gears and turned the millstones.

Head upriver just a short bit to the bridge site on your right. Here, rock relics of the bridge pinch in Duck River, which then shoots rapidly downstream. This location is known as Fishing Ford, the spot where Andrew Jackson crossed the river.

Continue in a riparian area, where wildflowers bloom throughout the summer. In other places, cedars thrive on the edge of limestone bluffs over which the trail passes. Side trails lead down to flat limestone outcrops along the river. Anglers may be seen

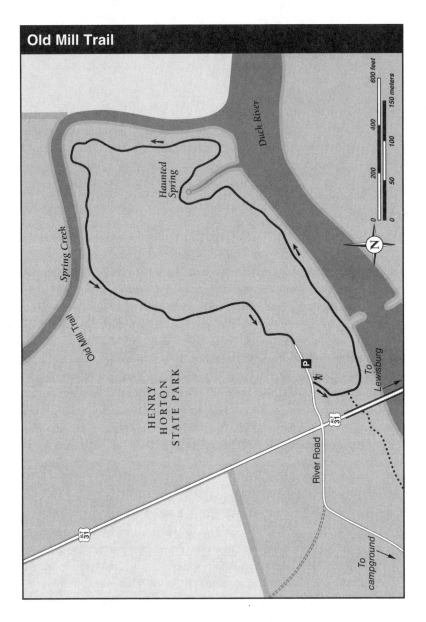

Old Mill Trail

down here, lazing away the day as the green Duck River flows downstream to meet the Buffalo River, which meets the Tennessee River. The trail turns away from the river as it passes over a few ravines via wooden bridges. The path is circling around Haunted Spring. Legend has it that a washwoman for the Horton family had her baby in a cloth sling as she was laundering at the spring. Her baby got away from her, fell in the river, and was never found, despite a massive search. Folks got to thinking the spring must be haunted to take away a baby so rapidly.

DISTANCE AND CONFIGURATION: 1-mile loop	ACCESS: No fees or permits required
DIFFICULTY: Easy	PETS: On leash only
SCENERY: River, river bluff, creek, woods	MAPS: USGS *Farmington;* at **tnstate parks.com/parks/about/henry-horton**
EXPOSURE: Mostly shady	FACILITIES: Restrooms, water at campground; picnic table at trailhead
TRAFFIC: Some traffic on weekends, otherwise quiet	CONTACT: 931-364-2222; **tnstateparks .com/parks/about/henry-horton**
TRAIL SURFACE: Wood chips, rocks, dirt	
HIKING TIME: 30 minutes	LOCATION: Chapel Hill

You'll briefly come near Duck River before turning upstream along Spring Creek, which is heavily grown up with beard cane along its edges. This rocky watercourse has bluffs of its own and may nearly dry out in summer and fall. Overhead, a young cedar thicket is reclaiming the village of Wilhoites Mill. Keep heading up along the creek. Imagine the post office, scales, and store that were once here, and the blacksmith shop that stood across the creek. Turn away from the creek along a wetland. Pass under a straight old woods road that was undoubtedly part of the village, and emerge in the trail parking area.

Nearby Activities

Henry Horton State Park offers hiking and excellent tent camping, while Duck River offers good fishing and family canoeing. A canoe livery very near the state park rents canoes and offers shuttle service.

GPS TRAILHEAD COORDINATES

N35° 35.612' W86° 41.755'

From Exit 46 on I-65, south of Nashville, head east on TN 99 for 4 miles to US 431. Turn right (south), and in 0.8 mile, continue east on TN 99 for another 7.4 miles to US 31 Alternate. Turn right on US 31A and follow it south 0.5 mile to Henry Horton State Park. Look left for a parking area just before US 31A bridges Duck River. This left turn is just across from the right turn into the state park campground.

44 Old Stone Fort Loop

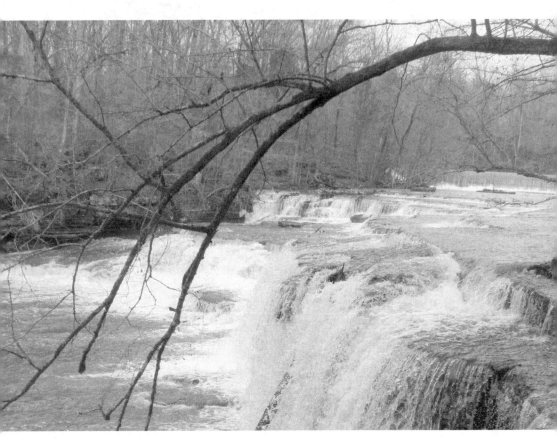

Close-up view of Blue Hole Falls on a chilly early-spring day

In Brief

This is one of Middle Tennessee's better hikes. You'll make a loop between the forks of Duck River, circling around a 2,000-year-old stone wall built by American Indians. Other features include several large waterfalls, rock bluffs, and remnants of milldams. An interpretive guide and state park museum enhance the experience.

Description

The narrow spit of land between the forks of Duck River is the setting for this hike, which melds American Indian history with the natural beauty of this fine state park. After leaving the museum, the hike circles an ancient American Indian enclosure marked by a stone

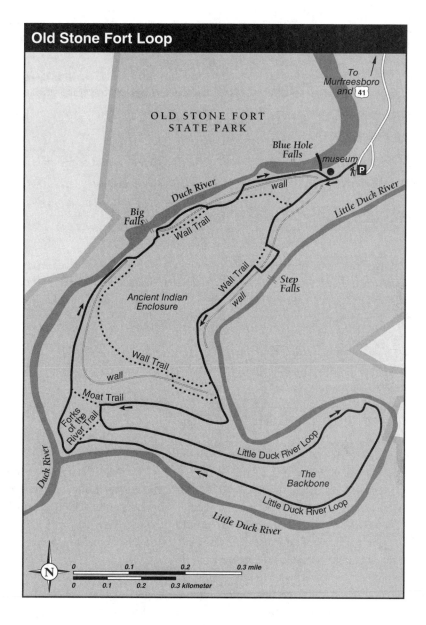

Old Stone Fort Loop

wall. Pass along Step Falls and the bluffs of Little Duck River before dropping into the Moat, an abandoned river channel. Climb along the narrow, rocky ridge of the Backbone before dropping back down to the water's edge to again meet Little Duck. Follow it to the confluence with the main Duck River. Climb past more of the stone wall and waterfalls of Duck River, along with old mills, before completing the loop.

After visiting the museum, begin your hike on Wall Trail. Stay left, looking at the 50-acre open field to your right. Because few artifacts were found, archaeologists have

DISTANCE AND CONFIGURATION: 2.6-mile loop	**ACCESS:** No fees or permits required
	PETS: On leash only
DIFFICULTY: Moderate	**MAPS:** USGS *Manchester*; at **tnstate**
SCENERY: High river bluffs, narrow rock ridge, riverside bottomland, waterfalls	**parks.com/parks/about/old-stone-fort**
	FACILITIES: Restrooms, water at museum
EXPOSURE: Mostly shady	**CONTACT:** 931-723-5073; **tnstateparks**
TRAFFIC: Moderate–busy	**.com/parks/about/old-stone-fort**
TRAIL SURFACE: Wood chips, leaves, rocks	**LOCATION:** Manchester
	COMMENTS: Visit the museum before you go on your hike.
HIKING TIME: 2 hours	

concluded that this enclosure was a ceremonial place and not a defensive or settlement location. Shortly, you'll reach a wooden walkway that heads over the wall and down to Step Falls on Little Duck below. Visit the falls and return via another boardwalk, returning inside the old wall. Cruise alongside the bluffs of Little Duck, peering down toward the water.

At 0.5 mile, you'll reach a concrete marker from 1966, which is used as a mapping point by archaeologists. The trail splits just past here. Turn left, descending on the River Channel Trail, also known as the Moat Trail. Veer right into a former riverbed of Duck River, before the watercourse bursts through a narrow ridge formed long before American Indians built the Old Stone Fort, which was developed over a 400-year period, from approximately A.D. 1 to A.D. 400. Beech and tulip trees grow where the water once ran.

Follow the Moat Trail to reach another junction at 0.7 mile. Turn left here on the yellow triangle–marked Forks of the River Trail, walking just a short distance to another junction. Turn left on the red square–marked Little Duck River Loop, and then climb onto the Backbone, a narrow rock ridge cloaked in mountain laurel. The Backbone widens a bit before the trail descends to the banks of Little Duck River. This area is rich with wildflowers in spring. Walk downstream alongside Little Duck amid lush woods. Bluffs form a rampart on the far side of the stream.

The bottomland gives way, as a hill on your right and the river on the left hem in the trail. The rocky, rooty track reaches another junction at mile 1.8. Stay to your left, now on the yellow triangle–marked Forks of the River Trail, and reach the confluence of Duck and Little Duck Rivers. Stand there and lament not having a fishing pole; then climb away to meet another junction. Stay left here on Red, Green, and Yellow Trail Access. Rise to meet Wall Trail again. Stay left again, heading up Duck River on a high bluff. Time has rendered the stone wall less noticeable here.

You'll soon reach a side trail leading left down to Big Falls, a massive cascade dropping over a rock face into a huge pool. A rock shelf stands beside the falls. Be very careful because the rocks are slippery around here. Look back away from the falls and you'll see large stone blocks, remnants of some mill operation. The path splits again—stay closer to the river—leading over a boardwalk and passing a more intact mill operation. This mill, the Whitman Mill, was built in 1852. Later, the Hickerson and Wooten Mill provided pulp for newspapers across Tennessee and the South, creating an entire community around the operation.

The final stop is the side trail to Blue Hole Falls, which is longer and wider than Big Falls. The trail takes you to the edge of the cataract, lending a look across its length as it spills over a ledge. Ahead is a dam built in 1963, before this was a state park. Shortly return to the museum and grab one last view from the observation platform above the museum. The questions you may have about the Old Stone Fort will probably require another visit to the museum after your hike.

Nearby Activities

Old Stone Fort State Park is one of Tennessee's most unsung destinations. Consider complementing your hike with a camping trip here.

GPS TRAILHEAD COORDINATES

N35° 29.173' W86° 6.133'

From Nashville, take I-24 East to Exit 111, Manchester. Head west on TN 55 for 0.8 mile; then turn right on US 41, heading north. Continue on US 41 for 1.7 miles and turn left into Old Stone Fort State Park. Follow signs to the Old Stone Fort and parking near the museum. The hike starts near the museum, 0.7 mile from the park entrance.

---

45 Short Springs State Natural Area Hike

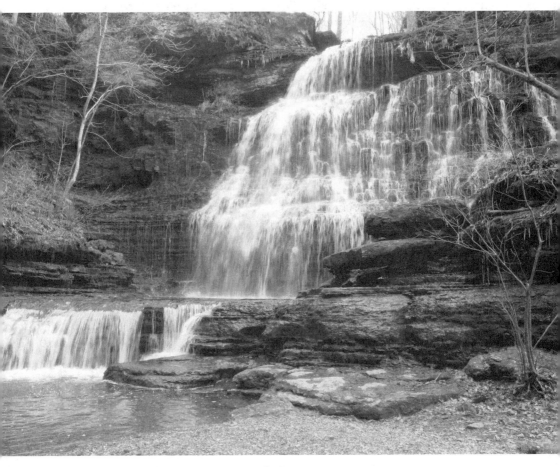

Machine Falls tumbles in tiers over stratified stone.

In Brief

This woodland in Coffee County is one of the best hiking destinations in Middle Tennessee. A well-developed trail system passes by clear streams that form waterfalls as they drop off the Eastern Highland Rim into the Nashville Basin. Dry, oak-cloaked ridges stand tall between these deep valleys where the water flows.

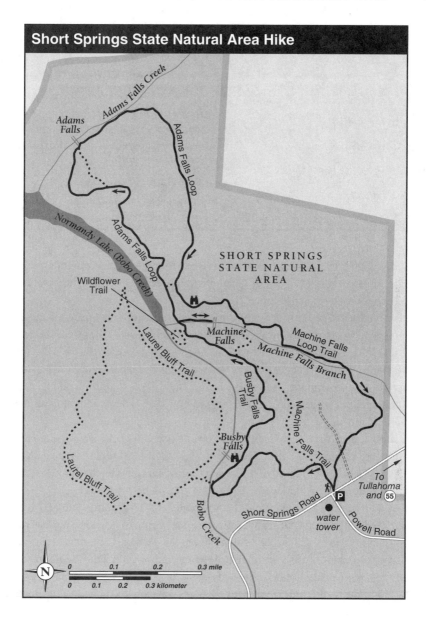

Description

Get here early to view all the waterfalls. This 420-acre state natural area includes rich woods, forest ravines, low cascades, springs, and big waterfalls, one of which I think should be in Tennessee's Top 10 Waterfalls list.

Thomas Busby saw power in the flowing water and built a mill here in the 1820s. After the mill closed, people began to believe that the translucent waters of these streams

DISTANCE AND CONFIGURATION: 3.2-mile loop with spur trails	**PETS:** On leash only
	MAPS: USGS *Normandy Lake;* at trailhead and at **tennessee.gov/environment /article/na-na-short-springs**
DIFFICULTY: Moderate	
SCENERY: Hardwood forest, waterfalls	**FACILITIES:** None
EXPOSURE: Shady	**CONTACT:** 615-532-0431; **tennessee.gov/environment/article /na-na-short-springs**
TRAFFIC: Moderate	
TRAIL SURFACE: Leaves, rocks	**LOCATION:** Tullahoma
HIKING TIME: 2.5 hours	**COMMENTS:** Be prepared to take waterfall photographs.
ACCESS: No fees or permits required	

possessed healing powers, and locals tried to attract tourists to the area. Today, the area is managed cooperatively by the city of Tullahoma, the Tennessee Valley Authority (TVA), and the Tennessee Division of Natural Heritage.

This circuit takes you by the three primary waterfalls at Short Springs, a major wild-flower preserve. From the trailhead, hike toward Machine Falls, but then veer away on Busby Falls Trail. Trace Bobo Creek to find the multiple levels of Busby Falls. You then rejoin Machine Falls Trail and descend to Machine Falls Branch. A spur heads up Machine Falls Branch, then seemingly dead-ends, but intrepid hikers continue along the water using stepping-stones and exposed rock to find 60-foot Machine Falls spilling between rock walls and forming a gravel beach.

The next feature to be seen is above an arm of Normandy Lake, via Adams Falls Loop and, of course, Adams Falls itself—a 25-foot Adams Falls tumbler that changes with water-flow levels, from a vertical dive to a slow seep. Start heading back toward the trail-head for a top-down view of Machine Falls; then you are back to the car.

Cross Short Springs Road to join the Machine Falls Trail. Immediately reach a trail junction. Head left, passing through hardwoods, and come to a second intersection and trail sign. This is where you hike left, downhill, on Bobo Creek Trail. At 0.4 mile, come to the concrete foundation of the former Boy Scout camp; then find the gorge of Bobo Creek. At this point, Laurel Bluff Trail heads left across Bobo Creek and makes a separate 1.2-mile loop you could add to your hike. Hike downstream, passing the cataracts of Busby Falls.

Come to Machine Falls Trail at 0.8 mile. Turn left and soon pass Connector Trail leading right. Keep straight on a narrowing ridgeline to descend steep wood-and-earth steps to reach Machine Falls Branch and another trail intersection. Wildflower Trail turns left and makes a short loop through a wildflower-filled flat. This hike turns right and heads upstream directly alongside Machine Falls Branch, heading for Machine Falls. The path seemingly dead-ends. However, look for placed stones and natural rock lead-ing along the right side of the creek. At high water this could be troublesome for hikers wanting to keep dry feet. Shortly reach 60-foot Machine Falls, an impressive small stream falls. Backtrack, then bridge Machine Falls Branch. Climb to intersect Adams Falls Loop at 1.2 miles. Keep straight along a steep wooded slope above the Bobo Creek arm of Normandy Lake.

At 1.7 miles, you will come alongside Adams Falls on your left. Ahead, criss-cross Adams Falls Creek several times, then turn away from the stream, curving south. At 2.3 miles, keep straight on the Machine Falls Loop Trail, then look for a spur leaving right and downhill to a partially obscured vista of Machine Falls. At 2.5 miles, meet the other end of Connector Trail, leaving right. Keep straight on Machine Falls Trail, crossing Machine Falls Branch at 2.8 miles. Start working uphill to reach the trailhead at 3.2 miles.

GPS TRAILHEAD COORDINATES
N35° 24.477' W86° 10.447'

From Nashville, head east on I-24 to Exit 111, Manchester. From there, take TN 55 West 4.7 miles to Belmont Road. There will be a sign here that reads TVA NORMANDY DAM. Turn right on Belmont Road and follow it 1.2 miles to Rutledge Falls Drive. Turn left on Rutledge Falls Drive and follow it 1.4 miles to reach a three-way stop. Turn right here, on Rutledge Falls Road. Follow it 2 miles to Short Springs Road. Turn left on Short Springs Road and follow it 0.8 mile to reach trailhead parking, on your left beneath a huge water tower. The trail starts on the far side of the road.

46 Smith Park Hike

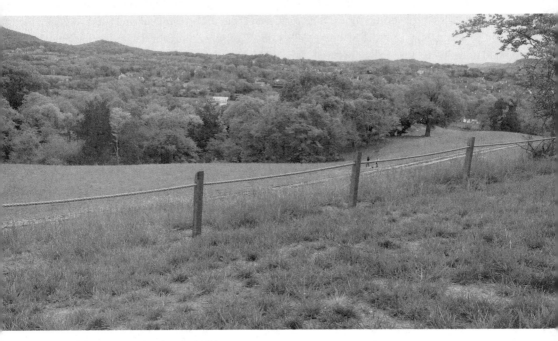

Looking across the Seward Hills

In Brief

This hilly loop hike circles through one of greater Nashville's newer preserves—Smith Park, located on the Ravenswood Mansion grounds, now public domain. Leave the trailhead parking area and ascend a knob to a wintertime view. From there, backtrack to resume the loop, dropping to a creek. Turn north in a mix of fields and woods before making a steep climb back into hill country. Wind through rocky woods, and then make your way back to the trailhead.

Description

Marcella Vivrette Smith Park is located on the grounds of the homeplace of one of Middle Tennessee's most prominent men—James Hazard Wilson II, a first-generation Tennessean. His grandfather Thomas Wilson emigrated from Ireland in the mid-1700s. At the age of 21, in the year 1821, James married his cousin Emeline Wilson, and the best man was none other than Sam Houston, the legendary Tennessean who later moved to Texas. When James and Emeline built their brick home in 1825, they named it Ravenswood after Houston, whose American Indian name was The Raven.

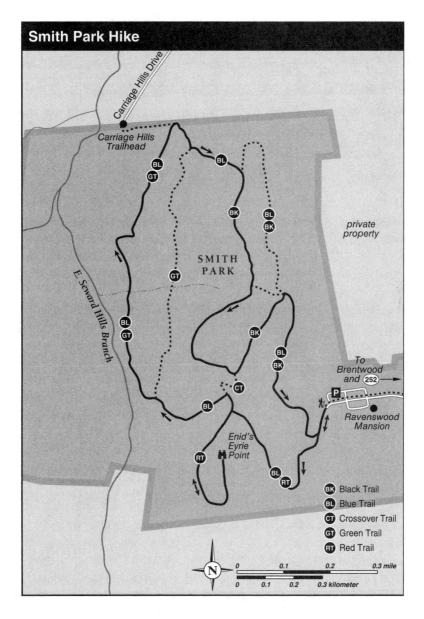

Smith Park Hike

Carriage Hills Drive

Carriage Hills
Trailhead

BL
GT

BL

BK

BL
BK

private
property

SMITH
PARK

GT

E. Seward Hills Branch

BL
GT

BK

BL
BK

To
Brentwood
and 252 →

P

Ravenswood
Mansion

CT

BL

Enid's
Eyrie
Point

RT

RT

BL
RT

BK Black Trail
BL Blue Trail
CT Crossover Trail
GT Green Trail
RT Red Trail

0　　0.1　　0.2　　0.3 mile

0　　0.1　　0.2　　0.3 kilometer

N

James Wilson began to build a plantation around the house, purchasing land from revenues generated growing cotton, eventually increasing his property to more than 1,000 acres. He continued to expand Ravenswood, becoming quite a wealthy man. He speculated in cotton properties, purchasing and operating plantations beyond the Volunteer State into Louisiana and Mississippi. Moving his product to market gave him the idea to acquire a steamboat line on the Mississippi River. Thus he not only made money growing cotton but also shipping it to market. Meanwhile, he fathered nine children, growing his family as propitiously as his business interests.

DISTANCE AND CONFIGURATION: 3.4-mile loop	**ACCESS:** No fees or permits required
DIFFICULTY: Moderate	**PETS:** On leash only
SCENERY: Ridges and hollows	**MAPS:** USGS *Franklin;* at **brentwood -tn.org/index.aspx?page=756**
EXPOSURE: Mostly shady	**FACILITIES:** Restrooms at trailhead
TRAFFIC: Busy on nice weekends	**CONTACT:** 615-371-0080; **brentwood -tn.org/index.aspx?page=756**
TRAIL SURFACE: Natural	
HIKING TIME: 2 hours	**LOCATION:** Brentwood

Things were going well. James invested in roadbuilding (Wilson Pike runs in front of Ravenswood) and later in railroads as they made their way to Middle Tennessee. Then the Civil War came. He spent thousands of his own dollars outfitting Confederate soldiers from the area. Happily, the mansion was not destroyed by the Yankees. In 1869 he passed away.

The mansion was continuously occupied but in an increasingly debilitated condition until 1961, when Reese and Marcella Vivrette Smith purchased the historic home and 500 acres still attached to the house, much of it part of the Seward Hills. With an eye for historic preservation, the couple restored the home but did have some non-historical amenities, such as an in-ground swimming pool. The couple raised their family there, but eventually the house was abandoned and sat vacant for 12 years until the three sons of Reese and Marcella began negotiating with the city of Brentwood about purchasing Ravenswood. It seemed a shame to let the property and house go. The city of Brentwood not only acquired the house but also 400 total acres of land, then restored Ravenswood. The plantation home is again the regal retreat it once was, and is now rented out for weddings, meetings, and special events.

You can see Ravenswood and the adjacent outbuildings from the trailhead. Leave south from the parking area, and quickly come to a trail intersection. Head left on the Blue Trail toward Enid's Eyrie Point. Climb sharply and quickly up a ridge cloaked in a mix of grasses and trees. Join the Red Trail at 0.4 mile. Head left here, climbing sharper than you might imagine possible in Middle Tennessee. Top out on the ridge at 0.6 mile, passing a huge oak en route. Join a grassy track left, reaching Enid's Eyrie Point at 0.7 mile. The views are more inspiring when the leaves are off the trees. Perhaps park personnel will fully clear the view by the time you hike here. Backtrack from the vista and rejoin the Blue Trail. Drop sharply, coming near a future park roadway (Smith Park is being developed in stages). Grab a view to the east of the Holt Knobs when you meet the Cross-over Trail at 1.1 miles. Cut through a gap and traverse a slope, descending toward the uppermost Harpeth River, which originates in the Seward Hills. Keep left on the Blue

Trail at 1.3 miles, as the Green Trail goes right. Pass near a pond, and then turn north and down the Harpeth Valley, though you can't really tell a river lies to your left; it seems more a creek at this point. Step over a stony, wooded tributary at 1.6 miles. Hike a mix of field and wood.

Reach an intersection at 2 miles. Here, a spur leads left to Carriage Hills. This hike turns right and climbs away from the valley up a cedar- and rock-covered hill that is quite steep. Pass the north end of the Green Trail at 2 miles and keep climbing on the Blue Trail. Reach another trail intersection at 2.1 miles. Turn right on the Black Trail—your climb isn't over yet. Finally top out at 2.3 miles, and then pass an old stone fence. Just ahead, a shortcut splits left. Stay right, descending to work around a wooded knob, still on the Black Trail.

At 2.7 miles, keep straight as you pass the north end of the Connector Trail. The Black Trail curves northeast to meet a four-way intersection. Turn right here, rejoining the Black Trail. Wind in and out of small hollows, bisecting fields and woods. Open onto a meadow, and complete the loop portion of the hike. The trailhead is visible below. Head downhill and finish the hike.

Nearby Activities

Smith Park has asphalt greenways in addition to the hiking trails. Ravenswood Plantation is available for special occasion rental. Future park developments will unfold with time.

GPS TRAILHEAD COORDINATES

N35° 56.820' W86° 46.392'

From Exit 67 on I-65, south of Nashville, take McEwen Drive east 3 miles to turn left on TN 252/Wilson Pike. Follow Wilson Pike 0.9 mile; then turn left into Smith Park. Follow the main park road past Ravenswood Mansion to the trailhead parking area.

47 Stones River Greenway of Murfreesboro

In Brief

The Stones River Greenway offers hikers a chance to enjoy both human and natural history in Murfreesboro. This paved path links earthworks and important sites from the Civil War's Battle of Stones River as it courses alongside the attractive Stones River.

Description

This greenway forms the link between various preserved portions of the Stones River National Battlefield. However, this trail is not just about Civil War history; it is also about recreation and appealing natural scenery along the Stones River as it flows through Murfreesboro. The nearly level trail leaves the old Fortress Rosecrans, then heads north, passing sites such as Braxton Bragg's Headquarters before ending near the old McFadden farm.

Start the walk at Fortress Rosecrans. What you see at the trailhead is but one side of what once was the largest enclosed earthen fortification built during the Civil War. The Union occupied Murfreesboro after the Battle of Stones River, which they won, but the main Union supply post was at faraway Louisville, Kentucky. General William Rosecrans ordered a fortified supply depot built here, so he could continue south toward Chattanooga and beyond. Rosecrans was following the Union strategy of driving a wedge through the Confederacy, ultimately leading to General Sherman's "March to the Sea." What you see today are the earthworks remaining from that supply depot. Walkways lead up to the earthworks and are enhanced with interpretive information.

Leave the parking area and head north along the paved and landscaped greenway. Fortress Rosecrans is off to your right. Soon you'll reach the iron trestle bridge over Lytle Creek. Here, the Lytle Creek Greenway goes right, and the Stones River Greenway goes left, staying atop a floodplain and crossing the Stones River. The Stones River Greenway is now on the west bank of the Stones River, where it will remain for the rest of the hike.

Look for an old milldam, over which the Stones crashes and splashes. Pass the Manson Pike trailhead, and walk underneath the old Nashville and Chattanooga Railroad—the rail line that prompted the Battle of Stones River. Reach the side trail to Redoubt Brannan at 0.7 mile. This trail leads left up to College Street and crosses the College Street Bridge back over the Stones River to reach the only remaining of four interior earthwork forts in Fortress Rosecrans. The College Street Bridge is where the Nashville Turnpike Bridge, which once connected Nashville and Chattanooga, stood.

Continue along the Stones River, passing a canoe launch for this popular paddling and fishing river. Silver maple, hackberry, and other moisture-loving trees line the

178

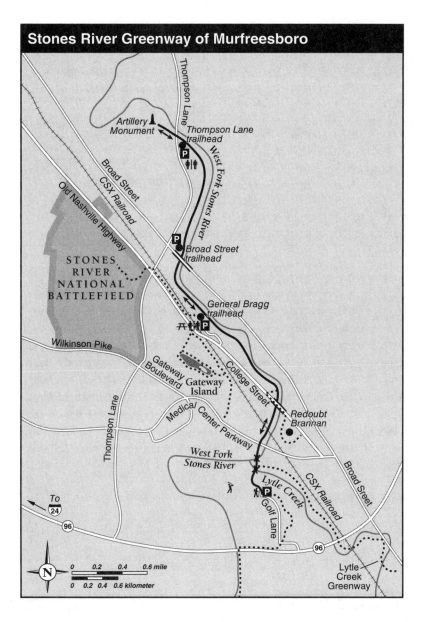

Stones River Greenway of Murfreesboro

watercourse. The canopy is often open overhead. Reach the side trail leading left to the General Bragg Headquarters site and trailhead at mile 1.6. This is the most developed trailhead and is where the spur greenway leads along College Street to reach Stones River National Battlefield near the Hazen Monument. It is from this spur greenway at the battlefield that you can access the Gateway Island trails.

Here, the Stones River Greenway leaves the floodplain for a rocky riverside bluff, offering a different river perspective. Pass the Broad Street trailhead at mile 2. Beyond

DISTANCE AND CONFIGURATION: 6-mile out-and-back	**PETS:** Must be on leash
DIFFICULTY: Moderate	**MAPS:** USGS *Walterhill* and USGS *Murfreesboro;* at **murfreesborotn .gov/DocumentCenter/View/370**
SCENERY: River valley, fort earthworks	
EXPOSURE: Partly shady	**FACILITIES:** Restrooms, water at General Bragg trailhead, halfway along trail
TRAFFIC: Fairly busy, but path is wide	**CONTACT:** 615-893-2141; **murfrees borotn.gov/index.aspx?NID=185**
TRAIL SURFACE: Asphalt	**LOCATION:** Murfreesboro
HIKING TIME: 3 hours	
ACCESS: No fees or permits required; daily, sunrise–30 minutes before sunset	**COMMENTS:** Path also connects to Lytle Creek Greenway and Stones River National Battlefield

here, the greenway becomes less used, as there are fewer access points. Shortly reach Harker's Crossing, the site where Union soldiers crossed the Stones, scouting and running directly into Confederate positions. This skirmish gave the Union important information on strategic Confederate emplacements.

The greenway is now back along the river, which flows in alternating riffles and pools. Continue as the greenway becomes busy again near the Thompson Lane trailhead, which you reach at mile 3. You can choose to turn around here, or continue 0.2 mile farther, passing a canoe launch and beneath Thompson Lane to reach the McFadden Farm Site and the Artillery Monument. Here, Union soldiers repelled a costly Confederate assault. From atop this hill it is easy to see how difficult it must have been for the rebels to cross the Stones River and climb the hill where Union cannons were firing away with deadly accuracy.

Nearby Activities

The Stones River Greenway is just one path in a greenway network of Murfreesboro. The Lytle Creek Greenway departs from the same trailhead as the Stones River Greenway, and the Battlefield Greenway connects the Stones River Greenway to the battlefield site.

GPS TRAILHEAD COORDINATES
N35° 51.133' W86° 24.753'

From Exit 78 on I-24, southeast of downtown Nashville, take TN 96 East 1.6 miles to Golf Lane. Turn left on Golf Lane and follow the signs 0.6 mile to Stones River Greenway.

48 Stones River National Battlefield Loop

In Brief

This loop hike traverses many sites at Stones River National Battlefield. See earthworks, cannon emplacements, memorials, and cemeteries interspersed into an attractive environment of woods, cedar glades, and fields. Before taking this hike, go into the battlefield visitor center to familiarize yourself with an important chapter of Middle Tennessee history.

Description

Explore the preserved portion of the battlefield where the Union and the Confederacy fought for control of the road and railroad connecting Nashville with states to the south. These lines were important for supplying troops on both sides. The Union strategy west of the Appalachian Mountains was to control the Mississippi River and drive a wedge into the Confederacy along the railroads of Tennessee and Georgia. With this second objective in mind, Union General William Rosecrans left his winter quarters in Nashville and headed for Murfreesboro, where the Confederacy's Braxton Bragg was stationed. With forces totaling more than 80,000 men combined, the two armies clashed during a three-day period, starting December 31, 1862.

The Confederates struck first, but their offensive was stopped. The two armies remained entrenched on New Year's Day, fighting little. But January 2, 1863, was a bloody day in American history, as a Confederate assault was pushed back by heavy cannon fire. Later, Braxton Bragg withdrew toward Chattanooga. The tactically indecisive battle resulted in more than 13,000 casualties. Today, you can walk amid much of the battle site, contemplating what happened on those fateful winter days. I recommend making this loop in winter to gain a better perspective of those troubled years.

Leave the picnic area on a mowed path, quickly entering a cedar thicket. Begin making a little loop on the Pioneer Bridge Earthworks Trail. At 0.2 mile, turn right, southbound on the Boundary Trail, in a mix of field and forest. Occasional limestone outcrops break the gravel path. At 0.3 mile, a trail leads left to the old auto-tour road, now a paved trail, where the Feds put up a line of defense to stop the initial rebel assault. Continue straight in a cedar forest, passing a second trail leading left to the road.

The Boundary Trail skirts around the battlefield boundary, passing a military park-survey marker at 1 mile. Another side trail leads left to the auto-tour road. The Boundary Trail continues, passing a marker indicating the site of the Blanton log house, just outside the park. Turn east here, nearing Wilkinson Road before turning into an area of cedars and rock outcrops. At 1.7 miles, head right on the Slaughter Pen Loop to an overlook of a sedate field, once the site of fighting so fierce it became known as the Slaughter Pen.

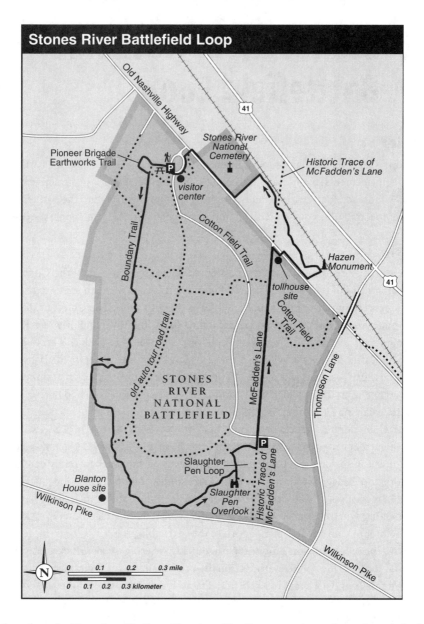

Stones River Battlefield Loop

Backtrack to the Boundary Trail, as Slaughter Pen Loop continues from the overlook to McFadden's Lane. At 1.8 miles, head right and soon reach the old McFadden's Trace. Turn north and follow the paved road on a designated hiker-only portion of the tour road.

At 2.2 miles, the paved Cotton Field Trail leaves right and links to the Stones River Greenway outside the battlefield. Keep straight along historic McFadden's Lane, and at 2.3 miles another paved portion of the Cotton Field Trail heads left toward the visitor center. Our hike keeps forward, then turns right along Nashville Highway, passing by a tollhouse site. Cross Old Nashville Highway here, at the white stripes painted on the road,

DISTANCE AND CONFIGURATION: 3.3-mile loop	**ACCESS:** No fees or permits
DIFFICULTY: Easy	**PETS:** On leash only
SCENERY: Forest and field	**MAPS:** USGS *Walterhill* and USGS *Murfreesboro;* at **nps.gov/stri**
EXPOSURE: Half sunny, half shady	**FACILITIES:** Restrooms, water, picnic area at visitor center
TRAFFIC: Moderate	
TRAIL SURFACE: Dirt, rocks, pavement, gravel, grass	**CONTACT:** 615-893-9501; **nps.gov/stri**
HIKING TIME: 2.5 hours	**LOCATION:** Murfreesboro

and pass through the split-rail fence on the far side of the road. Turn right, heading on a mowed path toward Hazen Monument. Take the paved path among large trees to reach the monument at 2.6 miles; it was erected in 1863 and is the oldest Civil War monument in existence. It states, "The blood of one third of its soldiers twice spilled in Tennessee. Crimson's the flag of the brigade and inspires to greater deeds." After Bragg retreated, Union men stayed in Murfreesboro for six months. While here, they interred their dead and built this memorial.

As you face the monument, look left for a path heading into the Round Forest, a site of major fighting. This location lies between what the battle was fought for—the railroad to your right and Nashville Pike to your left. Cross back over McFadden's Lane and keep forward, passing a marker noting where one of Rosecrans's aids was killed. Soon reach a stone wall, across which is the Stones River National Cemetery. Only Union soldiers, nearly half of whom are unknown, were buried in this still-active burial place. Walk along the wall back toward Old Nashville Highway and parallel the road, crossing Old Nashville Highway one last time to reach the park visitor center, completing the loop.

Nearby Activities

Stones River National Battlefield has a visitor center that offers a slide show and informative displays about this battle in particular, and the Civil War in general. Take time to enjoy the slide show, and consider taking the auto tour as well.

GPS TRAILHEAD COORDINATES

N35° 52.858' W86° 26.098'

From I-24 southeast of downtown Nashville, take Exit 74B to TN 840 East. Follow TN 840 East 1.9 miles, and take Exit 55A, Murfreesboro. Head south on US 41/70 South 1.7 miles to Thompson Lane. Turn right on Thompson Lane; then travel 0.3 mile and turn left to access Old Nashville Highway. Turn left on Old Nashville Highway, follow it 0.7 mile, and turn left into the visitor center. The hike starts at the picnic area near the visitor center.

49 Twin Forks Trail

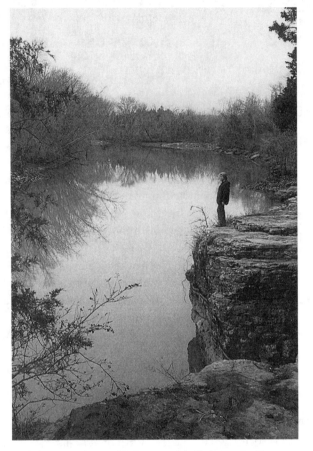

A hiker stands perched atop a bluff above the East Fork Stones River.

In Brief

This hike makes a loop around the East Fork Recreation Area on the upper reaches of Percy Priest Lake. East Fork refers to East Fork Stones River. The trail curves along the river, which nearly turns back along itself. Enjoy river bluffs and bottomlands in this slice of Rutherford County.

Description

This is just one segment of an 18-mile trail that winds along the banks of the East Fork and West Fork Stones River, connecting Nice Mill Recreation Area on the upper West Fork

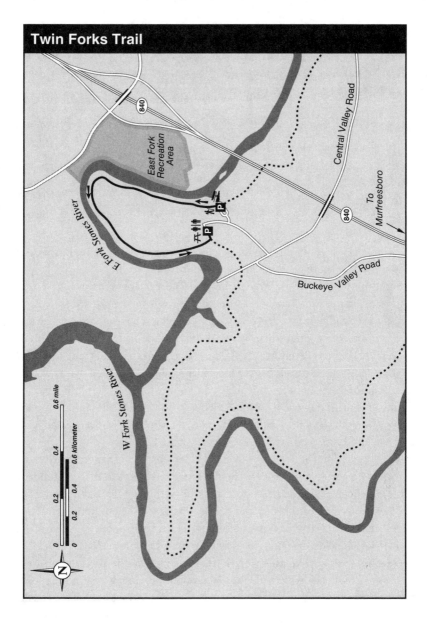

Stones River and upper East Fork Stones River near Walter Hill Dam Picnic Area. Trail users can pick up Twin Forks Trail at the above areas, as well as at the West Fork Recreation Area. The U.S. Army Corps of Engineers has an excellent map that will help steer you around Percy Priest Lake. Beware the trail's potential to flood out and be muddy in spring.

The East Fork Recreation Area is roughly in the middle of this segment of Twin Forks Trail. Though the path was built with equestrians in mind, hikers are welcome and frequently use the section around East Fork Recreation Area. This is a good place to get a

DISTANCE AND CONFIGURATION: 1.5-mile loop	**ACCESS:** No fees or permits required
DIFFICULTY: Easy	**PETS:** On leash only
SCENERY: Cedar bluffs, river-bottom forest	**MAPS:** USGS *Walterhill*; at **tinyurl.com/twinforkstrl**
EXPOSURE: Mostly shady	**FACILITIES:** Restrooms, water at East Fork Picnic Area
TRAFFIC: Moderate, busier on warm weekends	**CONTACT:** 615-889-1975; **tinyurl.com/twinforkstrl**
TRAIL SURFACE: Dirt, rocks	
HIKING TIME: 1 hour	**LOCATION:** Murfreesboro

taste of Twin Forks Trail, as you can make a loop hike out of it because East Fork Stones River makes such an acute bend it nearly doubles back on itself.

Start the hike by leaving the large parking area near the boat ramp; a little sign with a horse on it marks the path. Twin Forks Trail also leaves from the other side of the parking area. If you start heading toward TN 840, you are going the wrong way. If you are going the right way, you'll enter young brushy wood and reach some high limestone bluffs overlooking East Fork Stones River. At this point the river is dammed but still flows through a narrow channel. Little side trails lead to the cedar-studded bluffs and overlook points.

The East Fork embayment widens as you go downriver. The bluffs give way, and Twin Forks Trail drifts down to a bottomland hardwood forest. The path can be wet here, as it circles among the sycamore and maple trees. At 0.6 mile, a side trail leads right, to the river embayment. Bluffs stand tall on the far side of the East Fork.

Straddle the shaded and wooded margin between a field that covers the middle of the big river bend you are circling. This field is sown with crops to attract wildlife. In fact, bird boxes have been placed in the bottomlands for further wildlife enhancement. At mile 1.2, rise a bit from the bottomland into brushy young woodland. Soon you'll reach the East Fork Picnic Area, which has tables, grills, water, and restrooms. Big trees scattered in the grassy picnic area indicate that this may have been a homestead.

Recreation areas such as this were not always included in the long history of the Army Corps of Engineers, which was mostly about improving waterways for commerce. Involvement in navigation projects by the Army Corps of Engineers dates back to the early days of the United States, when rivers and waterways were the primary means of travel and trade. As the lands west of the original 13 states began to be settled, rivers became even more important because they were the only practical way of getting through the country's vast forests and mountains. Henry Clay of Kentucky lobbied for federal assistance in maintaining the navigability of such waters. Others thought it wasn't the job of the federal government. The Supreme Court settled it, ruling that the commerce clause of the Constitution enabled the feds not only to regulate navigation and commerce but also to make improvements in navigable waters. That decision gave birth to the Corps and its mission to maintain harbors, rivers, waterways, and, ultimately, trails and picnic areas.

Continue through the picnic area to reach the crumbling remnants of an asphalt road. Twin Forks Trail turns right here. You, however, turn left and follow the old road past a picnic shelter to the picnic parking area. Turn right at the parking area, and follow the road a bit to soon reach the trail parking area on your left.

Nearby Activities

The East Fork Recreation Area has a boat ramp, picnic tables, shelters, grills, and an added segment of Twin Forks Trail. The picnic area is closed in the cold season.

GPS TRAILHEAD COORDINATES

N35° 58.870' W86° 26.807'

From I-24 southeast of downtown Nashville, take Exit 74B to TN 840 East. Follow TN 840 East 4.8 miles to Exit 57, Sulphur Springs Road. Turn left on Sulphur Springs Road and follow it 0.6 mile to Buckeye Valley Road. Turn right on Buckeye Valley Road and follow it 2.9 miles to East Fork Recreation Area. Turn left into East Fork Recreation Area and follow the road 0.1 mile to the first right turn into a large parking area. As you are facing the water at the boat ramp, take the trail to your left.

50 Wild Turkey Trail

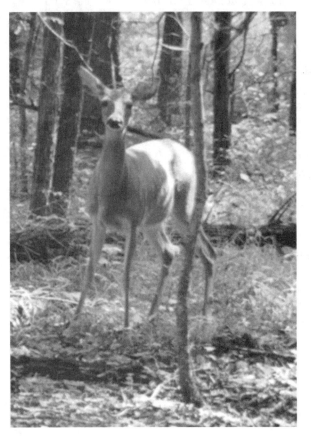

Deer are spotted with regularity at Henry Horton State Park.

In Brief

Henry Horton State Park's Wild Turkey Trail makes a loop through a cedar–oak–hickory forest that is fast reclaiming former farmland. You will see old fence lines and woods roads. Its low hills divided by intermittent streambeds make for some vertical variation as the path passes beside limestone outcrops and sinkholes. The mix of old fields and rising woods makes for good wildlife habitat not only for wild turkeys but also for deer.

Description

As we see more and more of Middle Tennessee getting eaten up by strip malls, roads, and subdivisions, it is heartening to see a slice of land return to its natural state. Such is the

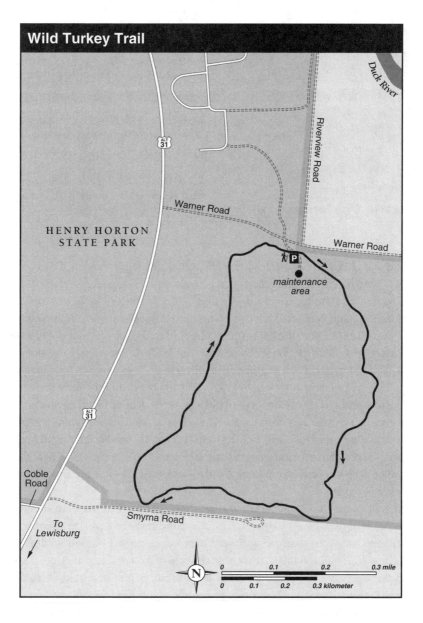

case in Henry Horton State Park, located just south of Duck River. The state of Tennessee owns the parkland, which it purchased from John Horton in the late 1950s. His father, Henry Horton, was a US senator and later governor of Tennessee from 1927 to 1933. Henry Horton married into the Wilhoite clan, which owned and operated a farm and mill on the banks of Duck River for more than a century. The community of Wilhoites Mill grew around this area, and there was once a post office, blacksmith shop, and general store. But times have changed in Duck River country since Henry Horton's day. You will

DISTANCE AND CONFIGURATION: 2.5-mile loop	**PETS:** On leash only
DIFFICULTY: Easy	**MAPS:** USGS *Farmington;* at **tnstate parks.com/parks/about/henry-horton**
SCENERY: Rolling, mostly forested country	**FACILITIES:** None at trailhead
EXPOSURE: Mostly shady	**CONTACT:** 931-364-2222; **tnstateparks .com/parks/about/henry-horton**
TRAFFIC: Moderate	**LOCATION:** Lewisburg
TRAIL SURFACE: Wood chips, dirt, rocks	**COMMENTS:** Trail may be closed during very occasional archery events at park archery range.
HIKING TIME: 1 hour	
ACCESS: No fees or permits	

get a firsthand glimpse of those changes while walking through what once was open farm country. The state park is letting the area regenerate at its own pace.

Leave the Wild Turkey trailhead, heading south, and descend into a hickory, maple, and cedar forest complemented with oak trees. Cedar trees love the limestone underpinnings of the soil here. Often the limestone emerges from the ground, as it does on many of the moss-covered outcrops you will see. The trail leads to a seasonal streambed that is more richly grown up than the thinner soil adjacent to it. In these depressions you are likely to find deer feeding or turkeys scratching. Turn away from the seasonal streambed and come to your first farm evidence—an old wire fence. Notice that the wooden posts of the fence are made of cedar, which resists rot well, assuring that these posts will be standing for a long time. Keep forward, looking right through the woods for a small pond. This was a farm pond meant for domesticated critters such as cattle or horses. These days, forest creatures like raccoons, foxes, skunks, and more make use of it. Look around for tracks on the edge of the pond.

The trail opens ahead and comes to a fast-disappearing clearing. Here, an old grassy farm road runs perpendicular to the trail. Look around at the edges of the clearing and see the brush and young trees growing here. These edges make for good wildlife feeding grounds as well. In not too many years, this clearing will completely disappear. Meander through shallow depressions and low hills, keeping an eye out for a sinkhole to the right of the trail. Here, a break in the limestone has allowed water to seep to a less resistant layer of rock and worn it away, causing the surface to collapse and forming a depression with no outlet for water. The lands around the state park and the Duck River basin are laced with sinkholes from which water runs underground and reemerges elsewhere. That is why some local farm ponds stay full rather than drying up—they are fed from underground. In contrast, some areas—like this sinkhole—won't hold water no matter what. Look for a couple of other sinkholes along the trail.

Curve around the state park boundary, now heading west. Look for shallow straight-line depressions in the forest that indicate other old farm roads. Returning north, the trail traces an old woods road that parallels a wire-and-wood fence. Meander over more low swales to emerge onto Warner Road. Turn right and walk a short distance back to the trailhead.

Nearby Activities

Henry Horton State Park offers not only hiking but also excellent tent camping. The nearby Duck River offers fishing and canoeing and has a fine picnic area along its banks. A canoe livery very near the state park rents canoes and offers shuttle service. For more information, visit **tnstateparks.com.**

GPS TRAILHEAD COORDINATES

N35° 35.005' W86° 41.348'

From Exit 46 on I-65, south of Nashville, head east on TN 99 for 4 miles to US 431. Turn right (south), and in 0.8 mile, continue east on TN 99 for another 7.4 miles to US 31 Alternate. Turn right on US 31A and follow it south 0.5 mile to Henry Horton State Park. After you pass over Duck River on US 31A, continue another 0.5 mile to Warner Road. Turn left on Warner Road and drive 0.2 mile to the trailhead, which will be on your right, near a park-maintenance building across from Riverview Road.

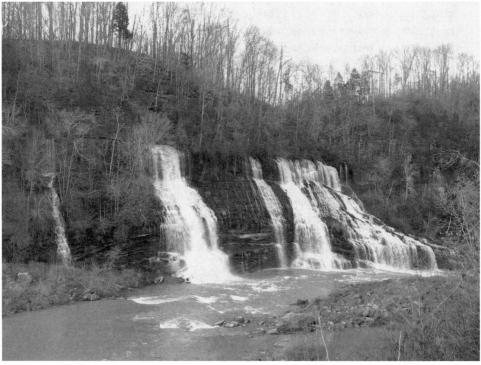

The waterfalls at Rock Island State Park are among the most impressive in Middle Tennessee (see page 205).

photographed by Jody Stickle

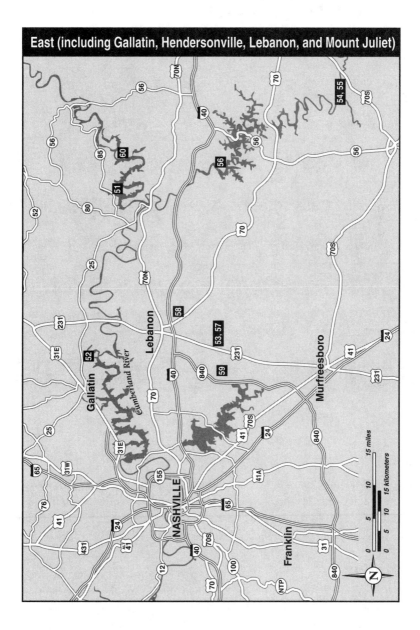

East (including Gallatin, Hendersonville, Lebanon, and Mount Juliet)

51 Bearwaller Gap Hiking Trail

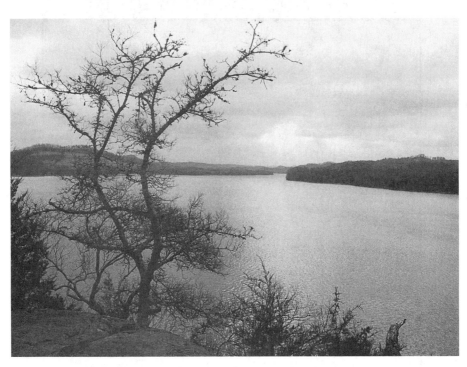

Hikers trekking the Bearwaller Gap Trail will be treated to views of Cordell Hull such as this.

In Brief

This is one of the finest paths in Middle Tennessee. It extends along the wooded and rugged shoreline of Cordell Hull Lake for more than 5 miles, passing waterfalls, old homesites, and rocky overlooks. It will challenge hardy hikers as it climbs and descends numerous times. Bring your stamina and ample time with you.

Description

Let's face it—some hikes are more rewarding than others. And the Bearwaller Gap Hiking Trail is one of the most rewarding hikes in Middle Tennessee. Why? It travels a considerable distance—5.6 miles one-way. Although it offers an old spring and other evidence of human habitation, it passes numerous natural features: rock gardens, overlooks, wet-weather waterfalls, and wildflowers in season. And it is physically challenging, traversing

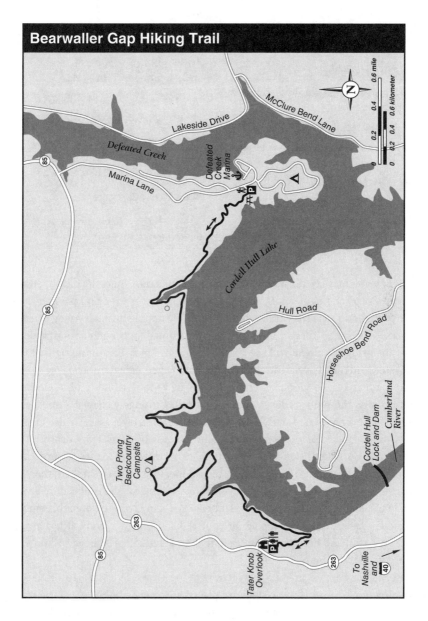

many ups and downs along the shoreline of Cordell Hull Lake. You can even backpack here because the trail has a designated backcountry campsite. Hikers can halve their distance, if confined by time and effort—the trail has parking areas at both ends, giving you the option of going either 5.6 or 11.2 miles. Be apprised that the Tater Knob Overlook trailhead is gated in winter.

This designated national recreation trail is named for the practice of bears "wallering" in moist, shady places during summer. Alas, no bears live in Middle Tennessee these

DISTANCE AND CONFIGURATION: 11.2-mile out-and-back	**PETS:** Must be on 6-foot leash
DIFFICULTY: Difficult	**MAPS:** USGS *Carthage;* at **tinyurl.com/cordellhullmap**
SCENERY: Wooded lakeshore and bluffs, numerous streams	**FACILITIES:** Restrooms, water at day-use area during warm season
EXPOSURE: Mostly shady	
TRAFFIC: Busy during warm-weather weekends	**CONTACT:** 615-735-1034; **www.lrn.usace.army.mil/Locations /Lakes/CordellHullLake.aspx**
TRAIL SURFACE: Leaves, dirt, rocks	
HIKING TIME: 6 hours	**LOCATION:** Carthage
ACCESS: Entrance fee required at Defeated Creek Recreation Area	**COMMENTS:** A backcountry campsite is located along the trail.

days, though you may see deer and wild turkeys on this trail. Start the hike by leaving the U.S. Army Corps of Engineers Defeated Creek Recreation Area and passing through a wooden fence beside the large trail sign. Immediately ramble through young brush before passing a second sign. Cross a wooden bridge and immediately enter a rock garden. Look just past the bridge, and you will see a small "window" in a rock to the right of the trail. Wind, water, and time have created this eye-catching geological feature.

The path is blazed along its entire length in yellow, white, and sometimes red. Ascend through the rock garden, appreciating other strangely shaped stones, and then switchback into a hardwood-and-cedar hillside to reach a level area. Cruise through flat woods. Cordell Hull Lake looms to your left through the trees, as it will nearly all the way to Tater Knob. Level out briefly before switchbacking downhill to turn toward an embayment of the lake; the going is slow on this steep slope. Pass a dry streambed, then a perennial stream, which has small waterfalls both above and below the trail. Curve around the embayment, passing a couple more streambeds. You can now see down this embayment into the main lake. Look for a spring on your right in brushy woods. It has a concrete-block catch basin, and just above the basin is the rocked-in springhead. A homesite was undoubtedly in the vicinity.

Enter a grassy area at mile 1.5. Stay left, with the brown sign and arrow indicating the correct direction. (More of these signs are placed at strategic points along the trail.) The Bearwaller Gap Hiking Trail now enters young woods and veers right, away from the lake. You'll reach a rock bluff that offers great southerly views of the dammed Cumberland River. Keep ascending on a narrow ridgeline to top out on a knob. Cordell Hull Lake is 400 feet below. Descend from the knob and pass two more rock-bluff overlooks before crossing an intermittent streambed.

Begin to skirt an embayment known as Two Prong. Curve around Ash Hopper Hollow, stepping over the streambed that creates the hollow, and come alongside a stone fence in this formerly settled area. Curve around the second prong of Two Prong and reach Two Prong Backcountry Campsite at mile 3. This area has flat spots for camping, as well as a covered spring, fire pits, a covered camping shelter, a picnic table, and an outhouse. Day hikers cutting their trip short can shoot for Two Prong as a turnaround point, making for a 6-mile out-and-back.

The trail climbs a wide roadbed to top out at mile 3.3, near a gate. Turn left here and make an easy and glorious walk along a level southbound ridgeline. Look for narrow, knife-edge sinkholes on the ridge. The easy walking soon ends, as the path travels past some odd-looking stacked-rock piles. Curve off the ridgeline, heading downhill to cross a rocky streambed at mile 4.1. Work around the small embayment with mossy walls of stone reaching to the waterline of Cordell Hull Lake. Shortly you'll pass an old homesite, where ivy grows wild and crosses the trail.

Beyond this point, the path ascends to come alongside a shoreline bluff. Cordell Hull Dam and other nearby bluffs are visible in the distance, and the lake lies far below. Just as you seem to near the dam, the Bearwaller Gap Hiking Trail veers abruptly right, away from the dam, and climbs toward Tater Knob. Reach the overlook restrooms at mile 5.5. Keep ascending past the restrooms to top out on a developed overlook. From here, hikers are rewarded with a sweeping panorama of Cordell Hull Lake, the Cumberland River, and the hill country through which it flows. From May through September, hikers can leave a shuttle car here. However, call ahead to make sure the overlook is open. Here are the directions to Tater Knob Overlook: From Exit 258 on I-40, east of downtown Nashville, take TN 53 North 4 miles. Continue as the road changes into TN 25 West 2.6 miles to reach TN 263 North. Turn right on TN 263 and follow it 3.6 miles to the overlook.

Nearby Activities

Defeated Creek Recreation Area has a campground, marina, picnic area, playground, and swim beach.

GPS TRAILHEAD COORDINATES
N36° 18.182' W85° 54.615'

From Exit 258 on I-40, east of downtown Nashville, take TN 53 North 4.3 miles, and continue as the road changes into TN 25. Go 6 more miles to reach TN 80. Turn right on TN 80 North and follow it 2.5 miles to TN 85. Turn right on TN 85 East, and follow it 3.6 miles to Defeated Creek Recreation Area. Turn right and follow the recreation area road 1.4 miles to a parking area on the right just before the campground entrance station. In winter, you must park over by the marina, beyond the campground entrance station.

52 Bledsoe Creek State Park Loop

In Brief

This loop hike traverses the perimeter of Bledsoe Creek State Park. Located near Gallatin, the park borders Old Hickory Lake. The trail offers lakeside walking, in addition to some hilltop walking through prime deer and wild turkey habitat.

Description

Bledsoe Creek is a small state park, and this loop makes the most of the scenic terrain included in this 164-acre preserve. Part of the scenery may well be wild turkeys. I don't know if it is just my luck, but wild turkey sightings have been part of every visit. It seems the turkeys are used to human contact, as they slowly but surely amble on after seeing people.

The beginning portion of the hike travels along paved all-access trails before picking up the natural-terrain Shoreline Trail. This path lives up to its name, as it traces the margin of land beside Old Hickory Lake. The loop then takes you to High Ridge Trail, which passes a homesite before climbing away from the shore and traversing a ridgeline 250 feet above Old Hickory Lake. High Ridge Trail then connects to Big Oak Trail, which curves past another homesite before dropping to the shoreline. Big Oak Trail gives way to Birdsong Trail and more paved pathways before completing the loop.

The first part of the loop can be confusing, so pay attention. Start the paved path to the left of the park office as you face it. Walk forward on the paved path, and soon you'll come to a four-way paved trail junction. Veer left here, and soon you'll reach a playground. Walk toward the water and then pick up the Shoreline Trail, marked with a sign. Old Hickory Lake will be to your right. The lake looks small here, but that is only because the park is located on the Bledsoe Creek arm of the long and large impoundment. Bledsoe Creek is located in Sumner County, once a rich hunting ground for American Indians and early settlers due to the abundance of natural salt licks in the area. Wildlife is still abundant in this state park: deer, turkey, rabbits, and even coyotes make Bledsoe Creek their home.

Watch for waterfowl as you take Shoreline Trail, curving as the shore curves. Straddle the wooded margin between the campground to your left and the lake to your right. Shortly, you'll reach the boat launch and fishing dock. Turn left, away from the lake, and head up the boat-launch parking area. Pick up High Ridge Trail in the upper-right corner of the parking area at mile 1. High Ridge Trail actually continues to parallel the shoreline, but the path is far above the water. Trace an old roadbed through a mixed hardwood and cedar forest, and then descend toward Old Hickory Lake. Keep an eye out for an old stone fence and level land to your left, marking a forgotten homesite. Of course, the folks who lived here looked down on a flowing Bledsoe Creek instead of the lake embayment.

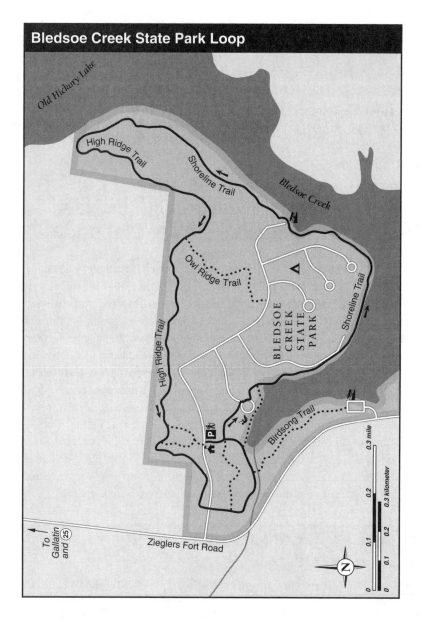

Bledsoe Creek State Park Loop

Span a ravine via wooden footbridge, and then climb a bluffline. Old Hickory Lake is still to your right, and soon you'll drop back to the lakeside. High Ridge Trail just can't make up its mind to stay high or low. However, it does offer open views of Bledsoe Creek embayment. Finally, High Ridge Trail makes up for its indecisiveness and climbs directly up the ridgeline with the help of wooden steps. A resting bench at the top of the hill looks appealing after that climb.

DISTANCE AND CONFIGURATION: 3.1-mile loop	**MAPS:** USGS *Bethpage* and USGS *Hunters Point;* at **tnstateparks.com/parks/about /bledsoe-creek**
DIFFICULTY: Easy–moderate	
SCENERY: Lakeside, forest	**FACILITIES:** Restrooms, water at park office
EXPOSURE: Mostly shady	
TRAFFIC: Busy during summer camping season	**CONTACT:** 615-452-3706; **tnstateparks .com/parks/about/bledsoe-creek**
TRAIL SURFACE: Leaves, rocks	**LOCATION:** Gallatin
HIKING TIME: 1.8 hours	**COMMENTS:** Bledsoe Creek State Park offers camping and water sports such as boating, fishing, and swimming. Picnic areas and playgrounds appeal to day visitors.
ACCESS: No fees or permits	
PETS: On leash only	

Soon you'll be walking along the park border, which is marked by a stone-and-wire fence. Skirt the border atop the ridgeline, topping out on a knob. Walk through young forest and reach a trail junction at mile 2.1. Continue forward, as a side trail leaves left toward the campground. You are now on Big Oak Trail, which soon slips off the ridgeline to the right, crossing a small spring branch on a pair of footbridges. An intact stone fence stands to the right. Climb away from this rich ravine into a cedar thicket. The campground office is visible to your left, but don't shortcut the loop—don't even think about it. Make one last climb of a hill, and then descend to another stream, which is crossed on a bridge.

Reach and cross the main park road to enter a cedar thicket in a flat, now back on paved pathway. This is Birdsong Nature Trail. Soon you'll reach a junction: Stay right here and cruise along a creek before curving past the park ball field. This flat is a wildflower haven in spring. Continue forward at the final paved trail junction and complete your loop. This final area may be confusing, but the park office is very near and can be reached in a matter of a few minutes no matter which paved paths you use.

GPS TRAILHEAD COORDINATES

N36° 22.602' W86° 21.372'

From Exit 95 on I-65, north of downtown Nashville, take TN 386 east 8.9 miles to take Exit 9 and merge onto US 31E North. Continue on US 31E North 7 miles to TN 25 East. Turn right on TN 25 East and follow it 5.3 miles to Zieglers Fort Road. Turn right and follow Zieglers Fort Road 1.4 miles to Bledsoe Creek State Park. Enter the park and leave your car near the park entrance station. The hike starts on a paved path on the right, just beyond the entrance station.

53 Cedar Forest Trail

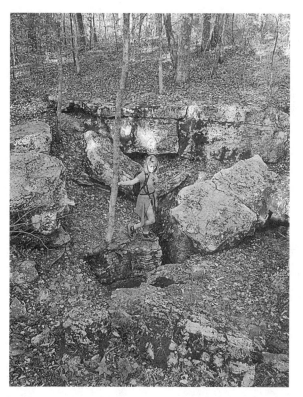

Rock-strewn sinks like this are a fascinating part of the Middle Tennessee landscape.

In Brief

This loop hike shows off the trees for which Cedars of Lebanon State Park was named. The trail passes through cedar woods but also penetrates hardwood forests on some of the state park's more hilly terrain, though none of the climbs are tiresome. Exposed rock gardens—areas with bleached limestone eroded into interesting shapes—punctuate the woods. The trail also passes numerous sinkholes of different sizes.

Description

The trail circles the northwestern section of Cedars of Lebanon State Park, a refuge that has become more important as metro Nashville pushes ever outward. What was quiet countryside on the outskirts of once sleepy Lebanon has become dotted with more and more homes.

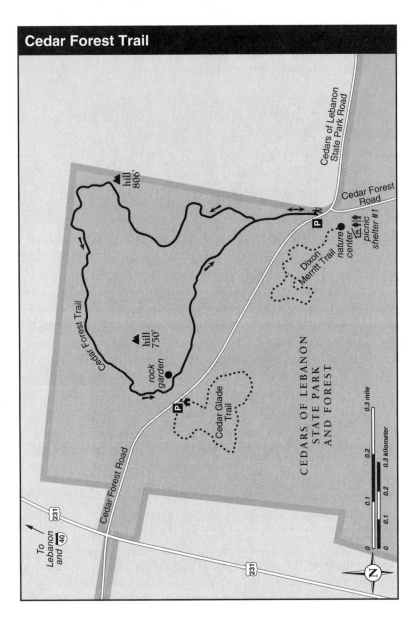

Cedar Forest Trail

Americans receiving land grants for their service during the Revolutionary War originally settled this area of Wilson County. When they arrived, these veterans found the land cloaked in vast cedar forests. These stands of cedar reminded them of the cedar trees of Lebanon referenced in the Bible and gave rise to the town's name. The settlers were determined to carve out a life in the cedars and used the trees on their farms for heating, to make shingles, and to build frames and chairs. Forest pockets were cleared for agriculture where the soil was thickest. Still, cedar was king of the county. Commercial timber

DISTANCE AND CONFIGURATION: 2-mile loop	**PETS:** On leash only
DIFFICULTY: Easy	**MAPS:** USGS *Vine;* at **tnstateparks.com /parks/about/cedars-of-lebanon** and at visitor center
SCENERY: Cedar and hardwood forest	
EXPOSURE: Shady	**FACILITIES:** Restrooms, water at visitor center; picnic area at trailhead
TRAFFIC: Busy on weekends	
TRAIL SURFACE: Dirt, rocks	**CONTACT:** 615-443-2769; **tnstateparks .com/parks/about/cedars-of-lebanon**
HIKING TIME: 1 hour	
ACCESS: No fees or permits required	**LOCATION:** Lebanon

operations came in the late 1800s, and they harvested the cedars for different purposes than farmers—for road boarding, telephone poles, fence rails, and pencils—items that could be sold in mass quantity. Cedar has always been the preferred material for pencils because its wood is soft. In fact, Cedar Key, off Florida's Gulf Coast, was denuded for the sake of pencils in much the same fashion as this area was.

After the harvest, farms sprung up in the vast clearings. More than 60 small farms were scattered throughout what would later become the 9,000 acres of state forest and park. The poor soil and limestone outcrops upon which cedars grow were terrible for growing crops; massive tree-clearing and poor agricultural practices led to erosion of the already marginal soil. In the 1930s, the federal government purchased these subsistence farms and turned the area into a demonstration project for forest reclamation and recreation management. One of the first assignments of the federal workers was to plant hundreds of thousands of cedar trees. Today, the forest has grown back, and you can enjoy the renewed woodland on this trail.

Leave the parking area by Picnic Shelter No. 1, and cross Cedar Forest Road to reach the Cedar Forest Trail. Turn left onto a crumbling paved road, and ascend. Turn left off the roadbed onto a singletrack footpath. At 0.2 mile, reach the actual loop portion of the trail. Turn right, skirt the state park border, and stairstep a moderate hill. Cruise alongside a rampart of rock on the hillside. A close look at the rampart will reveal subtle eroded shapes of rock carved over eons. Turn upward, cutting through the rampart to top out on a hill at 0.7 mile. The thicker soils atop this hill allow for the growth of hardwoods instead of cedars, creating more biodiversity. The trail turns left, gently drops down the hill, and begins to pass beside sinks and rock outcrops scattered beneath a forest of oak and maple. Curve around, passing a deep sink on your left. You can safely peer inside the hole here. Ahead, Cedar Forest Road is off in the distance to your right.

The trail twists and turns in a rock garden, so it is easy to see why the Works Progress Administration (WPA) of the 1930s used stone as its material of choice to construct the park buildings. The park lodge, picnic shelters, and other structures were built of native stone during this time. The impressive work of the WPA led to these buildings being added to the National Register of Historic Places.

Watch for a narrow, deep sink just beside the trail on the right. Descend, and then climb a bit to reach the end of the loop. Backtrack 0.2 mile on the crumbling asphalt road and complete the hike.

Nearby Activities

Cedars of Lebanon State Park has more than hiking trails. It offers a good campground, picnic areas, picnic shelters, a lodge, and cabins.

GPS TRAILHEAD COORDINATES

N36° 5.328' W86° 19.507'

From Exit 238 on I-40, near Lebanon, head south on US 231 for 6.4 miles to the state park entrance, on your left. Enter the park, get a trail map at the visitor center, and then drive a short piece to reach Picnic Shelter No. 1 on your right, 0.8 mile from the park entrance. Cedar Forest Trail starts on the left side of the road, opposite the picnic shelter.

---

54 Collins River Nature Trail

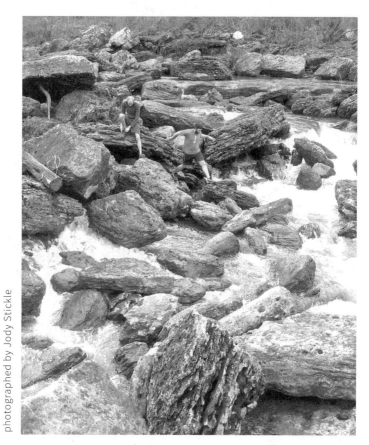

Hikers explore rocky river rapids of the Caney Fork River.

In Brief

This trail is not a nature trail in the classic sense. It has no interpretive signs. However, it does circle the attractive peninsula between Collins and Caney Fork Rivers. Water is never far away, and a practiced eye will discern old homesites scattered in the woods about this Tennessee state park trail. Nearby waterfalls add to the adventure.

Description

There are many ways to get to Rock Island State Park. However, none of them is easy. So relax, make an unhurried drive from Nashville, and enjoy a full day or more at this scenic gem of a getaway. Collins River Nature Trail may be the hook to get here, but you will see

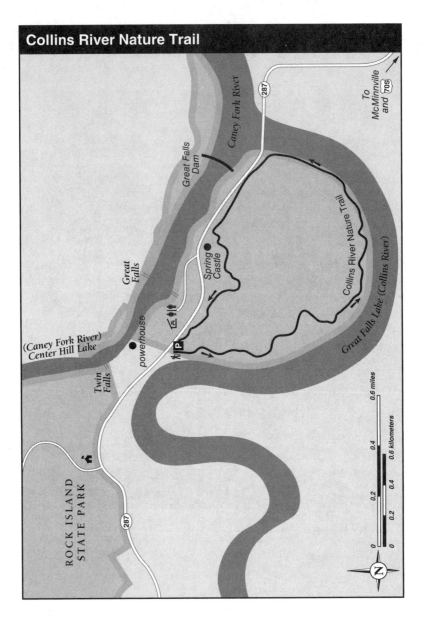

Collins River Nature Trail

there is more to behold than just this path. Swimming, boating, nature study, and camping may bring you back for more adventures. Eagle Trail, also profiled in this book, provides additional walking opportunities, as do the short paths to Great Falls and Twin Falls.

Because Collins River Nature Trail is just across the road from a powerhouse, it is not surprising that the path starts in an open field beneath power lines. These power lines are connected to the Great Falls powerhouse, which is fed by the Great Falls Dam. This dam was one of the Volunteer State's earliest hydroelectric projects. The Tennessee Electric

DISTANCE AND CONFIGURATION: 3-mile loop	**ACCESS:** No fees or permits required; daily, 7 a.m.–10 p.m.
DIFFICULTY: Easy	**PETS:** On leash only
SCENERY: Hardwood forest, big rivers	**MAPS:** USGS *Campaign;* at **tnstateparks .com/parks/about/rock-island**
EXPOSURE: Nearly all shady	**FACILITIES:** Restrooms, water at park office
TRAFFIC: Moderate, quiet during week	
TRAIL SURFACE: Leaves, dirt	**CONTACT:** 931-686-2471; **tnstateparks .com/parks/about/rock-island**
HIKING TIME: 1.7 hours	**LOCATION:** Rock Island

Power Company began constructing the dam in 1915 and completed it by late 1916. A one-unit powerhouse was erected adjacent to the dam. Ten years later, the dam was reconstructed, and a second power-generating unit was built. In 1939 Tennessee Valley Authority bought Tennessee Electric Power Company—a good thing, because the dam required extensive repairs in the mid-1940s. The dam and power plant have been in use since then, undergoing rehabilitation in the late 1980s. At that time, a road was built across the top of the dam. Before TVA took over the dam, homesteaders inhabited the peninsula between Collins and Caney Fork Rivers until the 1940s, when they were bought out and relocated. When you walk the trail, look for signs of these inhabitants.

Park at the open trailhead, and cross under the power lines. Shortly, you will pick up an old roadbed, which you will follow for most of the trail. This wide path makes for easy traveling. Furthermore, it has few hills, which makes the trail doable by nearly everyone. Soon enter the woods and veer right onto the old roadbed. The narrow ribbon of Collins River, backed up as Great Falls Lake at this point, lies to your right and will stay on your right the entire loop. A shortleaf pine and oak forest shades the trail.

Pass under a power line, also emanating from Great Falls powerhouse, and encounter a patch of yucca plants with stalklike leaves. The folks who once lived along this old dirt road likely planted the ancestors of these plants. A second, smaller power line opens the landscape and allows views of Collins River. The trail continues turning with Collins River toward Caney Fork, and the TN 287 bridge comes into view. The path veers right, off the roadbed, near Great Falls Dam, which is visible to the right through the trees.

After you backtrack over the old roadbed, keep your eyes open for the small Cunningham Cemetery to the left of the trail. The graves here have newer stones. The most prominent of the stones is that of John Cunningham, a veteran of the War of 1812. A dug well is near the graves, to the right of them as you face them from the trail. Stones have been laid in a circle down the well to keep its walls from caving in, but the bottom of the well has filled in. This is part of a homesite. I can only wonder which was here first—the graves or the well. It is unusual to have a well so close to a graveyard.

The next trail section reveals more homesite evidence. The forest is evenly aged. Small, level flats are scattered in the woods. Look for metal relics, such as old washtubs.

Spring Castle, located toward Caney Fork River, fed water to these homesteads. This circular building, still visible today from TN 287, captured water flowing off the bluff below and pumped it up to these residences. Great Falls Cotton Mill is located near the Spring Castle. This square brick building is pinched between TN 287 and Caney Fork River. It used waterpower to gin cotton but was in operation only a decade before floodwaters destroyed the waterwheel in the early 1900s. At this point, Collins River Nature Trail leaves the woods and emerges into a clearing broken by a large oak tree. The powerhouse is visible across the road. Make a short walk through the grass to complete the loop.

Nearby Activities

Rock Island State Park has an excellent campground, playgrounds, game courts, a boat launch, and other trails. Be sure to see Twin Falls and Great Falls while you are here. They are visible from the road over Great Falls Dam.

GPS TRAILHEAD COORDINATES
N35° 48.245' W85° 38.038'

From Exit 239A (Watertown) on I-40, east of downtown Nashville, take US 70 for 34 miles to TN 56 South in Smithville. Turn right on TN 56 South and follow it 9.3 miles to TN 287. Turn left on TN 287 North and follow it 10.8 miles, passing the main Rock Island State Park entrance on your left at 10.1 miles. Collins River Nature Trail is on the right on TN 287, across the road from the Great Falls Dam Powerhouse, less than a mile past the main park entrance.

---

55 Eagle Trail

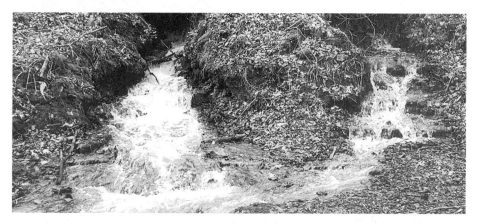

This trailside spring exhibits a strong flow.

In Brief

The sound of falling water is ever present along this path that traverses the gorge of Caney Fork River. Located below Great Falls Dam at Rock Island State Park, the trail connects two of the park's picnic areas and includes a rock scramble and river access at one end.

Description

This path packs a punch (and a half) into its short length set along a rugged portion of Caney Fork River. You will pass by smaller waterfalls to end near one of the state's most famous falls. How this falling water came to be is an unusual story.

In 1915 Tennessee Electric Power Company dammed the Caney Fork River, creating Great Falls Lake. The rising water level forced water from Collins River, above the dam, through caves that emerged on a rock face of Caney Fork River, below the dam. Since then, water has coursed through the caves. In some places, the falls are narrow drops with just a little mist. But others look like whitewater springs that burst forth from the mountainside. The granddaddy of all the falls makes a 300-foot-wide, 80-foot-long drop over a rock bluff into Caney Fork. This drop is known as Twin Falls. Great Falls, the lake's namesake, is actually a different cascade within the park boundaries. Eagle Trail takes hikers by some of these unique falls. However, some gorge-scrambling at the far end of the trail is necessary to reach Twin Falls. But don't hurry because the path has a few highlights along the way.

Start the trail at the Badger Flats Picnic Area. A sign indicates that the path was built under the guidance of a Boy Scout earning his Eagle Scout ranking. Pass the picnic-area restrooms and immediately enter a singletrack path. Caney Fork River, just freed from the Great Falls Dam upstream, flows clear green against a backdrop of tan and weathered

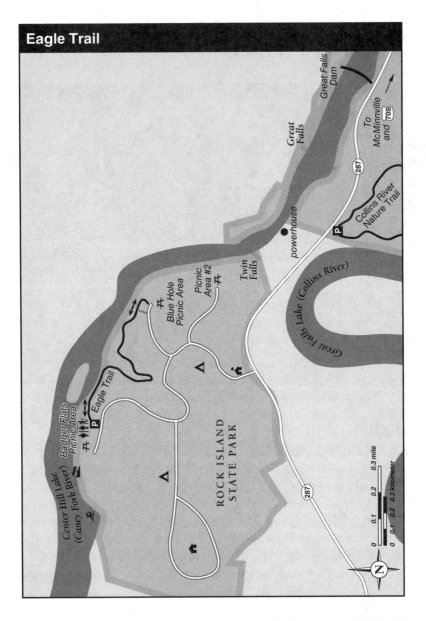

riverside bluffs. Overhead, hardwoods such as beech and hickory are sprinkled with some hemlock trees, less common in these parts. Look to your left for the last picnic table at Badger Flats. Then scramble off the path to your left and check out the first falls. Two cave openings spew water, which merges into one short stream and then falls from the riverside bluff into Caney Fork.

Ferns dot the ground beneath the forest as the trail twists among trees near the bluff's edge; an island splits Caney Fork River below. Past the island, Eagle Trail turns away from the river and climbs sharply as it works around a steep and narrow

DISTANCE AND CONFIGURATION: 1.7-mile out-and-back	**ACCESS:** No fees or permits required
DIFFICULTY: Moderate	**PETS:** On leash only
SCENERY: Riverside woods, bluffs, water galore	**MAPS:** USGS *Campaign;* at **tnstateparks .com/parks/about/rock-island**
EXPOSURE: Mostly shady	**FACILITIES:** Restrooms, water at trailhead
TRAFFIC: Busy on warm weekends	**CONTACT:** 931-686-2471; **tnstateparks**
TRAIL SURFACE: Dirt, rocks	**.com/parks/about/rock-island**
HIKING TIME: 1 hour	**LOCATION:** Rock Island

feeder-stream valley. Wooden footsteps aid the climb. You will hear the sound of falling water emitting from the small valley, but it is not coming from the intermittent creek at its bottom, not in this strange place. Let your ears lead you to a small bluff in the valley, where water is emerging through caves from Great Falls Lake, which is higher in elevation than the water-emergence location.

Keep circling around the steep cove to cross the intermittent streambed on a footbridge with handrails. Come to a roadbed roughly paralleling the river to reach Blue Hole Picnic Area. Another trail leads left from the picnic area down steps of wood, concrete, and metal into Caney Fork gorge. Here, numerous cave holes allow water to spray, foam, and descend toward the main river in multiple minifalls. Beyond the last steps, numerous paths wrangle among the water, rocks, and trees to reach the river below. The large, flat rocks along Caney Fork are great for sunning, swimming, and fishing.

Adventurous hikers and rock scramblers will keep upriver a short bit toward Twin Falls. Be careful, as the rocks can be slippery. The gorge is rich not only in falling water but also with wildflowers in spring.

Nearby Activities

Rock Island State Park has an excellent campground, playgrounds, and game courts in addition to a boat launch and other trails.

GPS TRAILHEAD COORDINATES
N35° 48.955' W85° 38.702'

From Exit 239A (Watertown) on I-40, east of downtown Nashville, take US 70 for 34 miles to TN 56 South in Smithville. Turn right on TN 56 South and follow it 9.3 miles to TN 287. Turn left on TN 287 North and follow it 10.1 miles, and then turn left into the park. The park office will be on your right after you enter the park. Continue 0.9 mile past the park office, and reach the Badger Flats Picnic Area on your right. Eagle Trail starts up the hill near the picnic area restrooms.

56 Edgar Evins State Park Hike

In Brief

This is one of Middle Tennessee's more challenging trails. Laid out by the Tennessee Trails Association, it offers a rugged hike on land managed by Tennessee State Parks and the Army Corps of Engineers. Set on the peninsula of Center Hill Lake, the hike, encompassing the Jack Clayborn Millennium Trail and the Merritt Ridge Trail, traverses formerly settled land, rocky ridges, lakeside bluffs, and lush wooded hollows.

Description

This is a challenging hike, no doubt about it. When the Tennessee Trails Association laid out this path, they wanted to take hikers to all of the highlights found on this hilly shoreline of Center Hill Lake. They met their goal. But to visit all these points and stay on public land, the trails had to make some serious twists and turns and ups and downs. The hike is worth every step, though. Be well rested and adventurous in spirit when tackling this trail, and you will have a good time.

This trail is known as a double balloon, which means it takes off, makes a loop, then heads on to make a second loop. Therefore, hikers can shorten their trek, walking only the first loop if they are short on time or energy, and still enjoy this path.

Jack Clayborn Millennium Trail leaves the park road and nears the shoreline before coming to the first loop, which passes by old stone walls and a homesite. The bulk of Jack Clayborn Millennium Trail heads out for a large peninsula jutting into Center Hill Lake. The topography is rugged out here, as the path heads up a narrow hollow and gains a ridgeline by a steep but short climb. It then rides the ridge before forming the second loop, where you can gain lake views from steep bluffs.

Start Jack Clayborn Millennium Trail by leaving the park road and heading down an old, gated woods road into a cedar copse alongside Center Hill Lake. The embayment to your right is ever narrowing as you come alongside a stone wall. Pass through the wall at 0.4 mile, reach a trail junction, and turn right. This is the beginning of the first loop. Cross a couple of intermittent streambeds and head up a wooded hollow to reach a small flat and a second trail junction. Piled rocks indicate this little area was once tilled. The trail to your left is your return route; stay right.

Head up the hollow, which is dominated by straight-trunked tulip trees. Where the hollow dead-ends, Jack Clayborn Millennium Trail ascends steeply to the ridgeline overlooking the hollow. Veer right and stay along the perimeter of Army Corps of Engineers land. The trail as a whole traverses both state park and Corps property, and oaks dominate the rocky ridgeline. Reach a high knob on the ridge at mile 1.7 and gain obscured lake views through the trees. An Army Corps of Engineers survey marker is planted into the ground here. Pass a seemingly out-of-place stone wall while descending from the

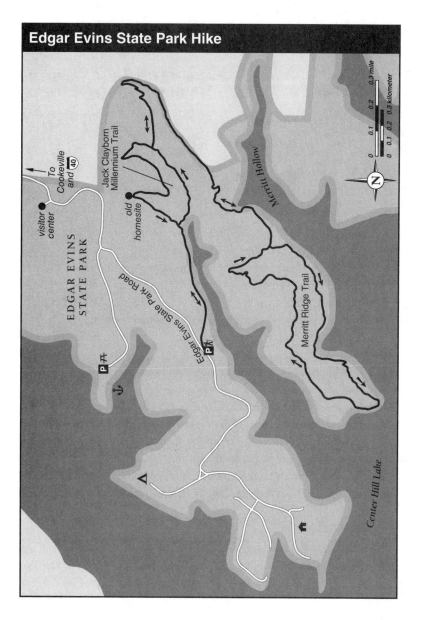

Edgar Evins State Park Hike

knob into a cedar thicket. Shortly, you'll reach a gap where a small, hand-dug pond lies next to a huge oak tree with widespread branches.

Millennium Trail descends to pick up an old woods road, then climbs to reach a gap and Merritt Ridge Trail at mile 2.4. Stay left here and begin paralleling the shoreline on a hillside of cedar and oak, shortly stepping over a crumbling stone wall. The main body of the lake lies to your left. Circle around a small embayment, and then climb to a backbone bluffline where you can peer out on the extent of Center Hill Lake between green cedar trees.

DISTANCE AND CONFIGURATION: 7.9-mile double balloon	**PETS:** On 6-foot leash
DIFFICULTY: Difficult	**MAPS:** USGS *Center Hill Dam*; at **tnstateparks.com/parks/about /edgar-evins** and at visitor center
SCENERY: Lakeside forests	
EXPOSURE: Mostly shady	**FACILITIES:** Restrooms, water at visitor center; picnic areas at state park
TRAFFIC: Moderate	
TRAIL SURFACE: Dirt, rocks	**CONTACT:** 931-858-2115; **tnstateparks .com/parks/about/edgar-evins**
HIKING TIME: 4 hours	
ACCESS: No fees or permits required	**LOCATION:** Silver Point

Descend along the bluffline to reach a cliff dropping into the lake. Here, Merritt Ridge Trail begins to curve back around the peninsula, and informal paths spur down to rocks at the water's edge. Cruise through thick woods, begin turning away from the water, and ascend the main ridgeline of the peninsula. Mostly angle up the ridgeline, until the final phase, which heads directly uphill to a gap in the ridge at mile 4.4. Once at the gap, turn left and climb on the nose of the ridge, passing another seemingly out-of-place stone wall. Meander atop the ridgeline for a half mile, and then drop again to complete this far loop at mile 5.

Return to the old roadbed and backtrack 1.7 miles to reach a familiar junction in the flat with piled rocks at mile 6.7. Turn right onto the untrodden portion of Jack Clayborn Millennium Trail, and trace an old farm road to shortly reach a homesite. Look for a rocked-in spring, a crumbled limestone block chimney, and foundations of an outbuilding atop the two-tiered flat. This site is a definite testimony to what was hardscrabble livin'. Ascend from the flat, and work toward a rock pile that was undoubtedly part of the homestead just passed. Descend along a woods road to reach another trail junction at mile 7.5. Once again reach familiar terrain, and backtrack the final 0.4 mile to complete the Millennium Trail.

Nearby Activities

Edgar Evins State Park is a good getaway for metro Nashville. It offers camping and cabins, hiking trails, and a marina. You can choose your level of comfort or challenge here. Also nearby are outfitters that rent canoes for floating Caney Fork River below nearby Center Hill Dam.

GPS TRAILHEAD COORDINATES
N36° 4.702' W85° 49.338'

From Exit 268 on I-40, east of downtown Nashville, take TN 96 South 3.7 miles to the park entrance. Keep forward, stopping in 1.5 miles at the park visitor center for a map. Continue another 1 mile and reach Jack Clayborn Millennium Trail on the left.

57 Hidden Springs Trail

In Brief

Hidden Springs Trail loops through a geologically interesting landscape full of rock formations and sinks, depressions in the land's surface that range from barely perceptible wooded dips to rock fissures deeper than they are wide. Other surface features are shady thickets of cedar trees that thrive in the thin soils and cedar glades, open meadowlike areas scattered in the forest. Overall, the hiking is easy, with little change in elevation.

Description

This is a good hike for those who want to learn about the relationship between the land and the plants that grow on it. Also, if you want to break into a longer hike, this is it. The terrain is nearly level, and the trail remains interesting throughout. Hidden Springs Trail is marked with white blazes painted on trailside trees. The path crosses numerous horse trails and some old roads, so stay with the blazes and backtrack if you're unsure.

Leave the parking area and cross Cedar Forest Road. Ahead is a trail sign. Hidden Springs Trail forks just beyond the sign. Take the right fork, as the path is easier to follow counterclockwise. It doesn't take long for the white-blazed path to pass by one of Middle Tennessee's signature features: a sink. These formations are caused by water erosion through caprock beneath the soil. Underground erosion continues, forming a cavern that eventually collapses and then becomes a sink. Sometimes these sinks are wide, bowl-like depressions; at other times they are deep and narrow. The numerous sinks you will see along this trail explain why there is very little permanent above-surface water here—it all runs into these sinks and into underground streams. Spur paths lead to many of the trailside sinks.

The level trail makes for easy walking among shagbark hickory, oak, redbud, and walnut, in addition to cedar trees, which sometimes grow in nearly pure stands. The forest here is broken with meadowlike clearings known as cedar glades. These clearings are natural rock gardens, albeit mostly flat, where the limestone rocks have pushed so close to the land surface that little or no soil can accumulate to allow for plant growth. In other places, where a thin soil does accumulate over the level rock gardens, the clearings may be covered with grasses or flowers. These cedar glades are a Tennessee treasure. In fact, 19 rare and endangered species of plants grow in this state and nowhere else.

Cross the first horse trail ahead. The bridle paths, identified with orange blazes, look more worn than Hidden Springs Trail, which only allows foot traffic. In places, it seems as if stones have been laid across the foot trail. Human traffic has eroded the thin covering of soil here, exposing the limestone underbelly of the forest. And sharp eyes will notice, on the left side of the trail, an old man-made pond that now functions as a wetland. Look for grasses barely covered with water.

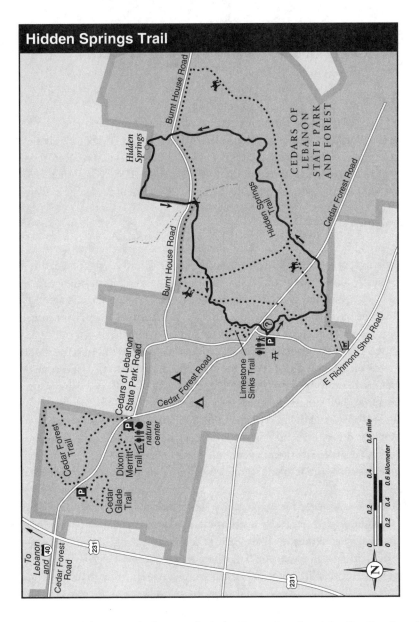

Hidden Springs Trail

Cross a second horse trail; then reach Cedar Forest Road at 0.8 mile. Continue forward to cross another horse trail. Notice how cedar trees grow differently depending upon their location: Those in open areas, or along the edges of glades, grow robustly green down to their base, and those in thickets (more competition for light) have dead branches at their sides and are green only at the top. More sinks are scattered throughout the woods.

The singletrack Hidden Springs Trail winds among thickets and glades. Old wire fences indicate that this was former pastureland—poor land composed mostly of rock and thin soil. Cross Burnt House Road at mile 2.5, and then reach a major sink on your right,

DISTANCE AND CONFIGURATION: 4.2-mile loop	**ACCESS:** No fees or permits required
DIFFICULTY: Easy	**PETS:** On leash only
SCENERY: Cedar forests and glades	**MAPS:** USGS *Vine;* at **tnstateparks.com /parks/about/cedars-of-lebanon** and at visitor center
EXPOSURE: Mostly shady	
TRAFFIC: Busy on weekends, moderate otherwise	**FACILITIES:** Restrooms, water at visitor center; picnic area at trailhead
TRAIL SURFACE: Dirt, rocks	**CONTACT:** 615-443-2769; **tnstateparks .com/parks/about/cedars-of-lebanon**
HIKING TIME: 2.2 hours	**LOCATION:** Lebanon

just past a wire fence beside the trail. Walk over to this huge sink, and you will see how limbs and brush have piled against the cave opening and the water inflow of the sink. You will also notice that the spot you are standing on is overhanging the sink.

Head up along the rocky streambed that flows into this sink, cross it, and look down into a narrow fissure that keeps the streambed dry. Cross back over the streambed and come to Hidden Springs, which is circled by a wooden fence. This spring is actually a dug well that accesses an underground stream, which is fed by all the sinks scattered in the woods. The relationship between these sinks and streams, both above- and belowground, is complex.

Turning away from the streambed, you'll see a rock face in the middle of the woods that would look oddly out of place anywhere but in this state park. Come near the park boundary in an area of larger hardwood trees, and then turn south on an old woods road to cross Burnt Woods Road again. Step over a dry streambed on a boardwalk. Pass through a pine plantation, and enter a hodgepodge of cedar glades, organized in a fashion designed only by Mother Nature. Rise into hill country growing up in hardwoods and broken with sinkholes aplenty. Pass two horse trails in succession, and then approach the Limestone Sinks Trail. A couple of side trails lead right, connecting to the Limestone Sinks Trail. Stay with the white blazes. Cross paved Cedar Forest Road, and reach the end of the Hidden Springs loop.

Nearby Activities

Cedars of Lebanon State Park is a great Nashville getaway. It offers a good campground, picnic areas, picnic shelters, a lodge, and cabins.

GPS TRAILHEAD COORDINATES

N36° 4.628' W86° 19.042'

From Exit 238 on I-40, near Lebanon, head south on US 231 for 6.4 miles to the state park entrance, on your left. Enter the state park, get a trail map at the visitor center, and continue 1.7 miles, turning right at a park picnic area just past the park swimming pool.

58 Sellars Farm State Archaeological Area

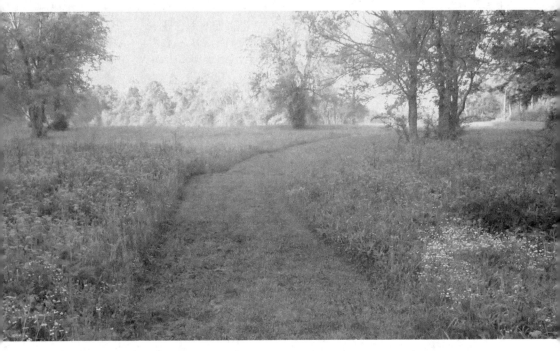

This path leads between the historic mounds and scenic Spring Creek.

In Brief

Take this rural hike through the fields and woods of a site harboring one of the best preserved aboriginal villages in the Southeast. The state archaeological area contains ceremonial and burial mounds, old walls, and palisades, and travels alongside scenic Spring Creek, with its sonorant shoals and stone bluffs.

Description

After the American Revolutionary War, a fellow named Nathaniel Lawrence claimed his land grant along the banks of Spring Creek in Middle Tennessee. He established a farm and passed it on to his descendants, one of whom was quite curious about the unnatural mounds and other earthen oddities on the property. In came archaeologist Frederic Putnam, who was the first to document and excavate this site, now recognized as one of the most intact

218

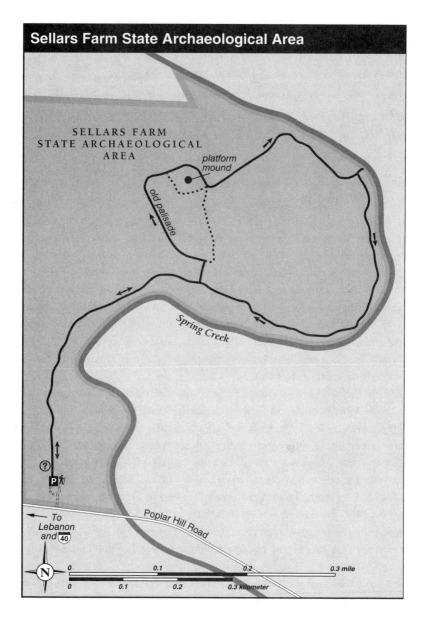

Mississippian Period villages in the Southeast. Later, James Sellars acquired the site and farmed parts of it himself, uncovering four stone human statues while plowing. The significance of the locale grew, and finally the state of Tennessee purchased the site in 1974 to preserve its aboriginal history. It took another 30 years for the former farm to be developed into the preserve we see today, where hikers and history buffs can gain glimpses into the past on a fascinating walking tour of a land occupied from around A.D. 900 to A.D. 1500.

DISTANCE AND CONFIGURATION: 1.5-mile loop	**ACCESS:** No fees or permits required; daily, 8 a.m.–sunset
DIFFICULTY: Easy	**PETS:** On leash only
SCENERY: Fields, woods, stream	**MAPS:** USGS *Shop Springs;* at trailhead kiosk
EXPOSURE: Half shady	
TRAFFIC: Very little, occasional tour groups	**FACILITIES:** None
	CONTACT: 615-885-2422; **tnstateparks .com/parks/about/long-hunter**
TRAIL SURFACE: Natural	
HIKING TIME: 1 hour	**LOCATION:** Lebanon

The aboriginals of the Mississippian Period picked a fine site for a village. First off, it is mostly circled by Spring Creek, which provided not only natural protection but also fish and freshwater mussels—and water. The flats in the bend were agriculturally rich soils as well. The aboriginals augmented the site with a defensive bulwark consisting of ditches and wooden palisades, made of the abundantly available and very sturdy cedar. Bastions were built into this wall around the site to thwart attacks. This is yet another example debunking the myth that pre-Columbian aboriginals were peaceful, noncombative societies. Fact is, pre-Columbian aboriginal groups warred with one another on a regular basis. It was part of their culture.

In addition to defensive vestiges of the village, there are also low burial mounds in addition to the most notable and easily recognizable platform mound, now topped with trees. The mound, 15 feet high, once had a building atop it, speculated to be the ruler's house or a council house. Other spots indicate the location of homes or other activity that is now lost to time. Of course, a lot of the area was used for agriculture; the farming of corn and having a steady food supply was a key development before a village could even be established. Previously, hunter/gatherer tribes had to be on the move, and therefore could not establish permanent settlements. Interestingly, around the year 1500, this village was abandoned for reasons unrelated to the arrival of Europeans on the American continent. After that, this region became a hunting ground of the Shawnee, Chickasaw, and Cherokee Indians.

The hike leaves the trailhead north from Poplar Hill Road. Stop at the informative kiosk and read up on the site. From there a doubletrack path leads into woods. Come near Spring Creek on your right before reaching the loop portion of the hike at 0.3 mile. Ahead is open field, and the main platform mound is visible in the distance. Head left on a mowed path through field to enter a line of woods along which you can see the remnants of the defensive palisades. Since this area was very rocky, the ditches and palisades were not plowed over like other areas of defensive works. Come to the main platform at 0.5 mile. It is clearly higher and not natural relative to the surrounding terrain. A grassy track circles the mound. Please stay off it to preserve the integrity of the site.

Beyond the mound, head east for Spring Creek. Soon sidle alongside the clear stream. Pools flow over gravel bars, creating little shoals. Across the way, stone bluffs rise majestically. It is easy to see why the Mississippians chose the site. Spur trails head down to the water. Continue along the creek, eventually rising out of the bottoms. Pass a stone wall from the 19th century. Rise back to farmland, completing the loop portion of the hike at 1.1 miles. From there, backtrack to the trailhead.

Nearby Activities

Sellars Farm State Archaeological Area is a satellite of Long Hunter State Park, which has trails galore.

GPS TRAILHEAD COORDINATES

N36° 9.909' W86° 14.566'

From Exit 239 on I-40, east of Nashville, take US 70 East 1.7 miles to turn left on Poplar Hill Road. Follow Poplar Hill Road 0.4 mile to reach the archaeological site entrance and parking area on your left.

---

59 Vesta Glade Trail

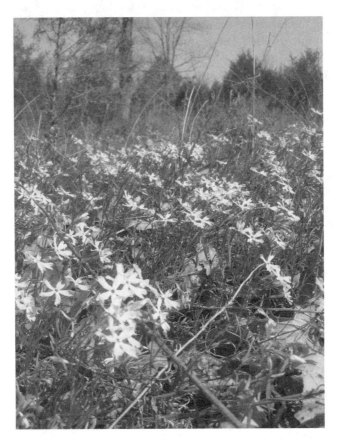

Phlox turn toward the sun.

In Brief

Vesta Cedar Glade is one of the newest additions to Tennessee's state natural area holdings. Located on the southern edge of Cedars of Lebanon State Forest in Wilson County, this little-visited area deserves more attention. It harbors parts of the globally rare cedar glades and offers wildflowers throughout the warm season, including the federally endangered Tennessee coneflower.

Description

For residents of Middle Tennessee, especially southeast of Nashville, cedar glades may seem a dime a dozen. In fact, the nearest town to Vesta Glade is called Gladeville.

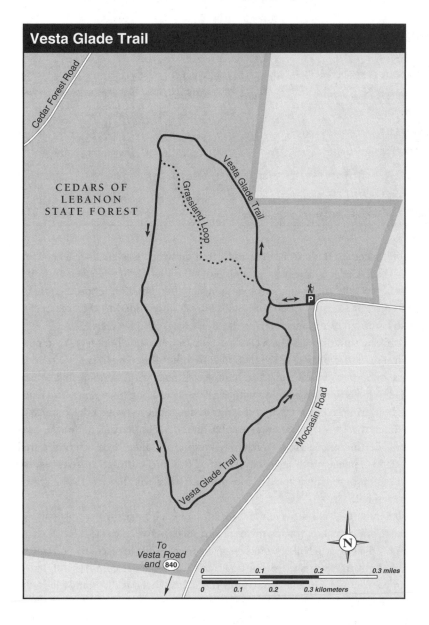

However, when you view cedar glades and barrens from a global perspective, these plant communities are extremely rare and occur nowhere else on the planet. Even on this preserve, parts of them are fenced off from the public to limit access and protect the resource. As greater Nashville grows, these glades become developed. So it is important that areas such as Vesta Cedar Glade be added to the Tennessee State Natural Areas program. It is also important that we visit such places, not only to personally appreciate them but also to let those who run these programs know their efforts are worthwhile.

DISTANCE AND CONFIGURATION: 1.8-mile loop	**PETS:** Must be physically restrained at all times
DIFFICULTY: Easy	**MAPS:** USGS *Gladeville;* at **tinyurl.com/vestacedarglade**
SCENERY: Cedar forests, open glades, hardwood forests	**FACILITIES:** None
EXPOSURE: Mostly sunny	**CONTACT:** 615-443-2768; **tinyurl.com/vestacedarglade**
TRAFFIC: Very light	
TRAIL SURFACE: Rocks and dirt	**LOCATION:** Lebanon
HIKING TIME: 1 hour	**COMMENTS:** There is a second, inner loop that can extend your hike.
ACCESS: No fees or permits required	

Public access to this special area and a trail on which to walk have been a long time coming. Vesta Cedar Glade was established after the Nature Conservancy bought a 90-acre tract in 1985 and sold it to the state, which then put it under protection. Later, 60 acres of adjacent Cedars of Lebanon State Forest were added to the area because that tract also harbored rare plants, making the area a total of 150 acres.

The hiking trail through Vesta Glade passes around some boulders, heading west on an old farm road to shortly reach a junction with foot trails going in either direction. Turn right here on a narrow foot trail. The blue-blazed path winds among sinks, then opens into a glade; this is the first junction with the Grassland Loop. Stay right. The fenced area you'll be bordering is the part that's off-limits to the public to protect the Tennessee cone-flower. Since the state natural area's establishment, Tennessee coneflowers have been found outside the fenced area, which may seem more open than where the trail goes, because land managers are aggressively using fire and cutting invasive vegetation to improve the natural habitat for the coneflower. Other wildflowers can be seen spring, summer, and fall.

At 0.5 mile, the trail turns left and reaches a bench beneath a sizable oak by an old farm road. Continue here, tracing the road as it slices between cedars.

Posts with arrows tell hikers which way to go, especially in places where vanishing but still visible farm tracks crisscross the trail. This was once agricultural land, likely cattle land, and you can see fence lines and farm relics. Just ahead is the point where the inner loop, the Grassland Loop, heads through more open areas back toward the trailhead.

The path stays mostly level, but its second half becomes more canopied. Continue tracing the old roadbed until mile 1.3. Here, the trail turns left onto a narrow track as a footpath in thick woods. Abruptly, the trail opens into a pair of gravelly glades. Watch for sinkholes bordering the trail beyond here. Just before completing the loop, pass a forgotten rock fence that likely bordered an old homesite. The settlers here probably never realized what a special place this was and that later the farm would be protected by the state for its outstanding features.

Nearby Activities

Cedars of Lebanon State Park is north of Vesta Cedar Glade. It offers picnicking, camping, and two other hikes featured in this book—Cedar Forest Trail and Hidden Springs Trail (see pages 201 and 215).

GPS TRAILHEAD COORDINATES

N36° 4.590' W86° 23.732'

From Exit 232 on I-40, east of Nashville, take TN 109 South 3.7 miles. Turn right on TN 840 West, and follow it 4.1 miles to Exit 67. Turn left (east) on Couchville Pike. At 0.5 mile, Couchville Pike meets McCrary Road. Continue straight through this intersection. Couchville Pike has now become Vesta Road. Continue on Vesta Road 1.3 miles; then turn left on Moccasin Road. Follow Moccasin Road 0.9 mile, and the trailhead will be on your left.

60 Wilderness Trail

In Brief

This trail, which is the most difficult trail in this guidebook, extends along rugged bluffs of the Cumberland River at Cordell Hull Lake. The trail, also known as Cordell Hull Lake Horse Trail, begins along the shoreline and climbs to the first bluff, only to descend to a steep, narrow hollow, then climb back out. This process repeats itself many times. However, your efforts are rewarded with vistas, solitude, and a waterfall along the way.

Description

This trail was a real surprise. The difficulty of the path was the big surprise, as it literally travels straight up and down these ravines. Its beauty was a mild surprise, with its far-reaching views from sheer bluffs cut by deep ravines cloaked in rich woods. Beauty has its price, though: Technically a horse trail, the path is also traveled by hikers and only lightly traveled by both groups. The U.S. Army Corps of Engineers trail map indicates that Wilderness Trail is a loop, but nearly the entire second half of the loop is on roads. Therefore, the trail is best enjoyed as an out-and-back hike. It is possible to put a car at the far end (directions are at the end of this description).

Begin Wilderness Trail by leaving the primitive Holleman Bend camping area on the path to the right as you face the lake. This trail quickly narrows as it passes through a brushy area. Forrester Hollow Lane is to your right. At 0.1 mile, the trail turns left, passing another large trail sign and a sign warning travelers, "Portions of the Wilderness Trail are extremely hazardous, steep, rough, and slippery." That is all true, but careful hikers have little to fear.

Climb just a bit, and then turn right on the far side of a rock wall built long before Cordell Hull Lake ever existed. Wilderness Trail parallels the wall, then angles up to meet the crest of a river bluff at 0.7 mile. The Cumberland River, now dammed but still a ribbon of water, lies to your left. The Salt Lick Creek embayment is visible through the trees. Continue east along the crest of the bluff as it climbs. Watch for a side trail leading right, cutting through another rock wall to your right. This trail leads into Forrester Hollow and is part of the Wilderness Trail loop.

Mile-marker signs of various ages and types are nailed to trees along the path. Soon, you'll pass mile marker 1, reach a high point on the bluff, and then descend to turn into an embayment at mile 1.5. Circle around the embayment to pass the stream flowing out of the hollow as it stairsteps into the lake. Pass another rock wall on the far side of the embayment. A little-used backcountry campsite lies trail-left before the path crosses a second streambed. Stay left; a private trail leads right. Keep the shoreline to your left, and shortly pass the brick and concrete remains of an old homesite.

Look to your right as the trail leaves the roadbed it has been following and veers up a hickory-and-oak-clad hill. Top out on the hill. A sheer bluff falls to the water below, and

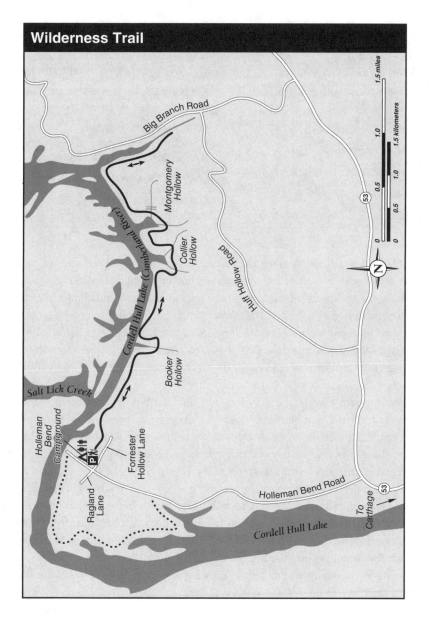

Wilderness Trail

another old stone fence runs away from the bluff. The descent from here is so steep you may be sliding on your backside before reaching the bottom. Climb just as steeply from the low point, topping out at mile 2.5. This next descent is more reasonable, but rocky, and leads to the two-pronged Collier Hollow embayment, the second major embayment along the trail. Again, circle around the embayment, stepping over a perennial stream. Open into a grassy clearing, and then step over an often-dry streambed—the second prong of the embayment.

DISTANCE AND CONFIGURATION: 12-mile out-and-back	**PETS:** On leash only
DIFFICULTY: Difficult	**MAPS:** USGS *Granville* and USGS *Gainesboro*; at **tinyurl.com/cordellhullmap**
SCENERY: River bluffs, small streams, thick woods	**FACILITIES:** Restrooms at nearby Holleman Bend Campground
EXPOSURE: Mostly shady	**CONTACT:** 615-735-1034; **www.lrn.usace.army.mil/Locations /Lakes/CordellHullLake.aspx**
TRAFFIC: Moderate	
TRAIL SURFACE: Dirt, rocks	**LOCATION:** Granville
HIKING TIME: 6 hours	**COMMENTS:** You can make the hike 6 miles with a car shuttle on both ends.
ACCESS: No fees or permits required	

Wilderness Trail curves along the lake and heads into another, smaller hollow, at mile 3.4. A sign advises equestrians to walk their horses through the sheer minigorge. The trail crosses the rocky streambed just above a wet-weather fall and climbs to circle back toward the main body of Cordell Hull Lake. Return to the bluffline and begin to circle into the two-pronged Montgomery Hollow embayment, crossing a clear stream at mile 4.1. Shortly, switchback out of the first hollow to reach a feeder stream forming the second prong of the embayment. Listen for the waterfall just upstream from the trail crossing. The low-flow cascade can be reached by simply walking up the creekbed.

Here, the path travels directly alongside the lake before once again climbing by switchbacks toward a high bluffline. The trail then abandons the switchbacks and heads directly uphill. The route is constricted, being confined to Army Corps of Engineers property. Good views can be enjoyed through the trees along the climb, and Smith Bend of the Cumberland River and the surrounding countryside can be seen. Top out in a grassy area at mile 4.9. The drop-off here is sharp, steep, and hundreds of feet in length.

Pass a sign advising equestrians to walk their horses before making a challenging descent; then ascend through a wooded ravine. Approach a barn on private property before dropping down a rocky bluff with mossy rocks and gnarled cedars. More views can be had while descending into the Big Branch embayment. The trail turns up the narrowing embayment in young woods before crossing Big Branch, which may be dry. Pass beneath a large sign indicating the Wilderness Trail at mile 6. At an intersection with Big Branch Road, a house is directly in front of you. To your left, downstream just a bit, is a spring and Army Corps property often used for camping. At this point, a car shuttle would be nice. Otherwise, you must backtrack.

If you choose to set up a car shuttle, back out of the Holleman Bend trailhead, the main trailhead, and return to TN 53. Turn left, north, on TN 53 and follow it to Big Branch Road. Turn left on Big Branch Road to reach the upper end of the embayment of Big Branch, where a large sign on the left, across from the aforementioned house, indicates the Wilderness Trail. If you have trouble finding this trailhead, just ask one of the friendly local residents, who will gladly point out the trail's end.

Nearby Activities

Holleman Bend primitive camping area, also known as Wilderness Campground, is at the trailhead. It offers primitive camping, with restrooms only.

GPS TRAILHEAD COORDINATES

N36° 18.800' W85° 47.732'

From Exit 258 on I-40, east of downtown Nashville, take TN 53 North and drive 4.2 miles, when TN 53 merges with US 70N East and turns right. Follow US 70N/TN 53 7.7 miles, and turn left to continue on TN 53 another 5.7 miles. Turn left on Holleman Bend Lane and follow it 2.6 miles to a four-way stop at Ragland Lane and Forrester Hollow Lane. Turn into the campground and parking area under the big sign that says WILDERNESS TRAIL. Wilderness Trail leaves east from the campground.

Appendix A: Outdoor Shops

Cumberland Transit West
2807 West End Ave.
Nashville, TN 37203
615-321-4069
cumberlandtransit.com

REI
261 Franklin Rd.
Brentwood, TN 37027
615-376-4248
rei.com

Cumberland Transit East
1900 Eastland Ave., Ste. 101
Nashville, TN 37206
615-942-8069
cumberlandtransit.com

Appendix B: Places to Buy Maps

Outdoor enthusiasts can find maps at the outdoor shops listed in Appendix A; an additional resource is below.

Map Sales and Services
1100 Lebanon Rd.
Nashville, TN 37210
615-242-3388
mapagents.com

Appendix C: Hiking Clubs

Tennessee Trails Association

tennesseetrails.org

The Tennessee Trails Association is the oldest hiking club in Middle Tennessee. The group has more going on all over the state than most hikers have time to enjoy. It is a sponsor of the Cumberland Trail and does much work in building and preserving trails and managing the wild areas of the Volunteer State.

Nashville Hiking Meetup

meetup.com/nashville-hiking

This Internet-based hiking group, thousands of hikers strong, is a great place to meet fellow hikers and go hiking, among other fun activities. They hike not only greater Nashville but all of Middle Tennessee and beyond.

Index

About the Author

Johnny Molloy is a writer and adventurer based in Johnson City, Tennessee. His outdoor passion ignited on a backpacking trip in Great Smoky Mountains National Park while he was attending the University of Tennessee. That first foray unleashed a love of the outdoors, which led the native Tennessean to spend more than 3,500 nights backpacking, canoe camping, and tent camping over the past three decades.

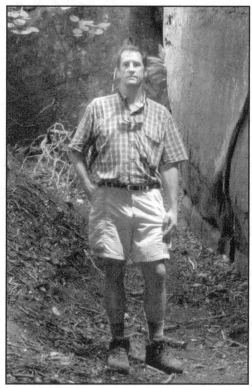

Friends enjoyed his outdoor adventure stories; one even suggested he write a book. He pursued his friend's idea and soon parlayed his love of the outdoors into an occupation. The results of his efforts are more than 60 books and guides. His writings include hiking, camping, and paddling guidebooks; comprehensive guidebooks about specific areas; and books of true outdoor adventures throughout the Eastern United States.

Though primarily involved with book publications, Molloy writes for various magazines and websites and is a columnist and feature writer for his local paper, the *Johnson City Press.* He continues writing and traveling extensively throughout the United States, endeavoring in a variety of outdoor pursuits.

A Christian, Molloy is an active member of First Presbyterian Church in Johnson City, Tennessee. His wife, Keri Anne, accompanies him on the trail and at home. Molloy's non-outdoor interests include reading, American history, and University of Tennessee sports. For the latest on Johnny, visit **johnnymolloy.com.**

DEAR CUSTOMERS AND FRIENDS,

SUPPORTING YOUR INTEREST IN OUTDOOR ADVENTURE, travel, and an active lifestyle is central to our operations, from the authors we choose to the locations we detail to the way we design our books. Menasha Ridge Press was incorporated in 1982 by a group of veteran outdoorsmen and professional outfitters. For many years now, we've specialized in creating books that benefit the outdoors enthusiast.

Almost immediately, Menasha Ridge Press earned a reputation for revolutionizing outdoors- and travel-guidebook publishing. For such activities as canoeing, kayaking, hiking, backpacking, and mountain biking, we established new standards of quality that transformed the whole genre, resulting in outdoor-recreation guides of great sophistication and solid content. Menasha Ridge continues to be outdoor publishing's greatest innovator.

The folks at Menasha Ridge Press are as at home on a white-water river or mountain trail as they are editing a manuscript. The books we build for you are the best they can be, because we're responding to your needs. Plus, we use and depend on them ourselves.

We look forward to seeing you on the river or the trail. If you'd like to contact us directly, join in at www.trekalong.com or visit us at www.menasharidge.com. We thank you for your interest in our books and the natural world around us all.

SAFE TRAVELS,

Bob Sehlinger

BOB SEHLINGER
PUBLISHER